HAIR TODAY,
GONE TOMORROW?

HAIR TODAY, GONE TOMORROW?

DEALING WITH UNWANTED BODY HAIR

Dr Antonia Bradbury

Thorsons
An Imprint of HarperCollins*Publishers*

Thorsons
An Imprint of HarperCollinsPublishers
77–85 Fulham Palace Road,
Hammersmith, London W6 8JB

Published by Thorsons 1992
1 3 5 7 9 10 8 6 4 2

A catalogue record for this book
is available from the British Library

ISBN 0 7225 2623 7

Printed in Great Britain by
HarperCollinsManufacturing Glasgow

CONTENTS

Introduction   ix

Chapter 1: **Attitudes to Body Hair**   1
Introduction   1
The 'Normal' Distribution of Body Hair   3
Attitudes towards body hair   5
Physical and sexual significance of body hair   6
Non-sexual attitudes towards women's body hair   10
Tribal attitudes towards body hair   11
References   12

Chapter 2: **How Hair Grows**   13
Introduction   13
Types of hair   14
The structure, growth cycle and transformation
   of hair and follicle   18
The pattern of women's hair growth   29
The regulation of women's hair growth   33
Medical definitions of excess body hair   37
Seeking medical help for excess body hair   38
Medical treatment for women with excess body hair
   and no underlying disease   46
Underlying diseases that cause excess body hair   50

Chapter 3: **Temporary Methods of Hair Removal**   52
  Introduction   52
  Disguise   54
    Bleaching   54
    Make-up   58
  Depilation   58
    Shaving   59
    Trimming   65
    Depilatory creams   65
    Abrasives   69
  Epilation   70
    Plucking and tweezing   70
    Electric epilating devices   73
    Threading   75
    Waxing   75
  References   89

Chapter 4: **Electrolysis: A Permanent Method of Hair Removal**   90
  Introduction   90
  Methods   91
    Galvanic electrolysis   93
    Thermolysis   95
    'The blend'   96
  Commencing electrolysis   96
    The Salon   97
    The Epilation Machine   97
    The Electrologist   99
  The effectiveness of electrolysis   102
  Causes of high regrowth rate   104
  Initial temporary clearance of hair   115
  Estimation of time and cost for specific areas of hair   117
  Contraindications to electrolysis   120
  Problems and side-effects   124

Self-electrolysis   127
Electrolysis in the USA and Australia   129
References   131

Index   133

Dedicated to E. Morton Bradbury

INTRODUCTION

The physical characteristics of our bodies change in many ways as we grow and age: our height and shape, the distribution of fat and muscle, and the development of wrinkles are just some examples of how we change; the distribution and quality of our body hair is yet another. In men and women the changes in body hair can bring distress or joy, depending upon the social conventions they live with.

The social pressure on women to remove their body hair is considerable. All forms of the media exhort the ideal of the perfect (hairless) woman. It is not surprising that women, finding themselves hairier than this ideal, begin to worry about what is happening to them. In fact, women are often asked by their relatives, friends or partners to seek medical advice about treating their 'hair problem'; worried mothers frequently take their daughters to see their GPs.

As a doctor I have been consulted by women with these worries, some of which I have shared myself during a period of my life. After reading books and articles, I became clearer in my own mind of the psychological and medical issues involved in the problems of body hair. In doing so I realized that much of this information was not available to most women, and that a great deal of their suffering was unnecessary and could be alleviated by a book of this kind.

This book starts with a brief insight into the reasons why we feel the way we do about our body hair, then goes on to describe all aspects of hair growth, and concludes with the different ways of dealing with unwanted hair. These include psychological, medical and cosmetic advice, and should help guide you towards the best way of dealing with your body hair. If you choose to remove it, I have described all the methods available, as well as their advantages and disadvantages.

This book will have served its purpose if by the time you have finished reading it you feel less troubled with your body hair, however you decide to deal with it.

1

ATTITUDES TO BODY HAIR

Introduction

All women have different distributions of body hair, ranging from fairly hairless to quite hairy. Some of these women will feel that their body hair is quite acceptable in society, whereas others will feel that they have far too much (a very small minority will feel they have too little, but this is another issue). The reason that women feel *any* particular way about their body hair is the pressure put upon them by our society (in many different ways) to conform to a particular image of the 'acceptable woman'. For example, all eye colours are equally acceptable in this society as being feminine, as is the height of a woman (except for absolute extremes). Different hair colours, however, conjure up different images of womanhood, each one of which is nevertheless equally a woman: blond hair suggests sexy or innocent, black hair suggests passionate or vampish. Similarly, different body shapes conjure up different images of woman: a full body with wide hips and big breasts suggest a Mother Earth image, whereas slim hips and tiny breasts suggests youth and innocence.

If we compare these attitudes to the images conjured up by body hair, there is a difference: the ideal woman should have a perfect pubic triangle and a beautiful head of hair, plus or

minus underarm hair (depending on the society); any
deviance from this is regarded as unfeminine and even masculine; the more you deviate from this image the more likely
you are to be regarded as looking 'like a man'. For example
moustaches, leg hair, nipple and lower back hair, all of
which are fairly common in women (see page 30), are not
regarded by society as feminine characteristics, but rather as
masculine ones. This means that society has taken normal
female variants and labelled these variants as 'non-womanly'
or masculine. It would be equivalent to regarding all women
above the height of 5ft 8in as having a masculine characteristic.

This is very different from having an unattractive characteristic, for example (and I am aware that all of the following
characteristics can look attractive in the right setting) a big
nose, crooked teeth or knobbly knees. These just have the
label of 'unattractiveness' put upon them, but body hair has
the label of 'masculinity' attached as well. This is a much
stronger label, and carries with it a greater social stigma.

It is not surprising then, that from the bombardment of
the media, articles and expectations from all aspects of society, we build up in our minds an image of a 'normal'
woman: if we differ from this towards being what is regarded as 'masculine', we become less self-confident as women,
secretly ashamed of the offending characteristics, and even
too embarrassed to talk about them. This is what has hap-
pened with body hair: all women that deviate too much from
the image of a 'normal' woman are ashamed to reveal their
situation, and so each woman believes that she is alone with
her own problem – to reveal it would mean showing the
world a painful, intimate secret which no one else shares. So
these women hide the hair or remove it secretly, not knowing that at least 20 per cent of the female population are
doing just the same. Have courage, you are not the only one.

The 'Normal' Distribution of Body Hair

The socially accepted 'normal' distribution of body hair in women is very different from 'natural' body hair distribution. The most obvious difference is that natural body hair is far more abundant than socially accepted body hair. Another difference is that the distribution of natural body hair is a creation of biology and evolution, whereas socially acceptable body hair is created from centuries of attitudes, culture and fashion. Thus natural body hair has hardly changed through history, and the only changes in distribution and quality are seen in different races. The distribution of socially accepted body hair, on the other hand, changes with time and fashion (what is accepted now as 'normal' is different to what was accepted as normal 100 years ago), and with culture (what is acceptable to British society is not acceptable in Italy, for example). To a greater or lesser extent throughout history and culture, however, the socially accepted female has been less hairy than the natural female.

Society's original reasons for preferring a female with little body hair have mainly been forgotten; with time society has become conditioned to preferring what it sees, and for centuries the hairless female has been a built-in cultural preference. This preference is, however, open to modification by several social forces.

The strongest force is fashion. Fashion dominates women's attitudes about appearance, behaviour, lifestyle, and regarding body hair; fashion and its propaganda make it very clear to the public what the 'ideal woman' should be. So, for example, bushy eyebrows are now completely accepted as part of the female image (thanks to Brooke Shields), and recently a delicate covering of fine leg hair has also become more acceptable (look at the actress Daryl Hannah).

An increasingly powerful social force however, is the
Women's Movement (obviously this force is intimately associated with fashion; the direction and' way in which women
are changing will guide and change fashion). Women are
now seeking economic, political and sexual independence
from men, and the attitude of 'accept me as I am' is developing in women and being carried throughout society. Never
before have we had so much freedom to do as we want and
to be as we wish to be. Just as men have had this kind of
freedom for many years (although admittedly they are not
completely free from these kinds of social pressures), so are
we beginning to taste it. It is up to us to try and express our-
selves as we really are, difficult though it may be, and in
doing so, slowly lead fashion in the same direction.

There is a small example that makes this point quite clearly: the attitudes and behaviours towards hair on the head.
Like body hair, head hair has had symbolic labels and attitudes attached to it through history, and was until recently
mainly under the influence of fashion and the idea of the
dependent female, i.e. hair-styles that were regarded as feminine. Nowadays head hair is very much a product of the attitudes of the new independent woman; hair-styles are first and
foremost practical and easy to maintain, and only secondly
must they be 'feminine'. We have lead the way to this
change and fashion has followed us. We can do this in relation to attitudes about our body hair, too.

If there was a time in history when a woman was most
free to choose what to do with her body and her body hair it
is now. More than ever, the choice of how to lead her life
regarding physical appearance is hers. Of course it will take
time to change centuries of attitudes, but step by step it is
possible, and it has to be initiated by us.

Attitudes towards Body Hair

Through the ages and different cultures, removal of body hair, in both males and females, was the accepted norm in society. Exactly when and why this initially developed is unknown, but it is known that this practice started independently in different cultures, at different times and for different reasons. There are several reasons for removing body hair that have been described through history, and as I have mentioned, although these reasons formed the basis for our present attitudes, they have mainly been forgotten:

HYGIENE
It was believed, and in some cultures still is, that body hair was unhygienic (in both men and women) because it traps sweat and dirt. Thus it was considered better removed.

RITUALS AND RELIGION
Body hair has played a role in tribal rituals for centuries, and from these have stemmed many of the present-day religious rites; body hair either being preserved completely (Sikhs), hidden (Christianity and Judaism), or shaved (Muslims), according the beliefs of the particular religion.

AESTHETICS
A smooth body was perceived as more aesthetically pleasing than a hairy one (in both men and women). This probably started as an attempt on the part of humanity to distance itself from its hairy animal friends. How many Renaissance paintings or Classical statues have you seen that depict the body as hairy?

SEXUAL DIFFERENTIATION
Men and women are different but complementary beings, and for centuries societies have tried to accentuate these dif-

ferences (physical, intellectual, emotional and psychological). The pursuit of distinct male and female characteristics has lead to the few physical ones being exploited and exaggerated to an extreme. For example, in men height and body muscle are significant signs of 'masculinity', whereas for women fine features and smooth skin are signs of femininity.

FASHION

At some time during civilization (most noticeably during the reign of Louis XIV, in 17th-century France, and since) the aristocracy had free time and money on their hands, and in order to appear as though they were doing something, they invented, amongst other pastimes, the art of fashion. During the course of time this gradually seeped its way down through the classes and has now infiltrated all aspects of our lives. Most of all, however, it has affected women and is the cause of the obsession with physical appearance. The attitudes, and the consequent habits of females, towards their body hair have been, and continue to be, moulded by fashion.

Physical and Sexual Significance of Body Hair Through History

Around the time of the ancient Egyptians and Greeks it was believed that body hair was unhygienic and aesthetically unappealing; this attitude was later adopted by the Romans. In men and women both, all body hair was removed — young boys, however, were regarded as objects of ideal beauty, and were required to keep their pubic hair, as this hair was particularly admired.

In the Middle East, long before the Roman Empire and since, Judaism was one of the established religions in which homosexuality and bisexuality were prohibited. Men and women had distinct sexual roles, and body hair removal in women was commonplace. This practice continued in the Middle East for centuries.

Over in Europe, at the end of the Dark Ages and the beginning of the Middle Ages (around 1000 AD), it was a time of sexual freedom; the Church and its dogma were far from established and the land was full of myths about wizards and sorcerers. Men wore their hair long with unkempt beards, and women wore theirs loose or in plaits; body hair was left natural and nudity was not regarded as shameful.

During the Crusades, there was a rediscovery of the civilizations of the East, and with it a discovery of the custom of the removal of body hair in women. This custom arrived in Europe at a time when the Church was starting to enforce its dogmas and sexual taboos upon the people, especially upon women.

By the 13th century, the Church was well established and the sexual freedom of the Middle Ages had been converted to a sexual neurosis (a triumph of the Church!). It was believed that female hair (but also women in general) was a sexual provocation, to be covered or removed, and women spent the next few centuries working hard at proving their worth and trying to 'appear' as chaste as possible.

For part of the 16th century in France there is evidence (a report by a certain Jean de la Montagñe) that it was considered elegant for women to shave both their upper and lower body. However, by the beginning of the 17th century, Catherine de Medici, Queen of France, put a stop to hair removal in females; it was kept for use on hysterical women only. Catherine de Medici was an obese, narcissistic and domineering woman, but I wonder if she also had abundant body hair?

In 18th-century Europe, fashion in the courts of the great courtesans reached an obscene peak. Women were wearing their head hair in massive head-dresses requiring wire, plaster, wool and other materials to be kept in place, decorated with feathers, lace and models of fruit, animals, birds, battle scenes and whatever else took their fancy. Their faces and bodies were powdered white to give a porcelain look, and body hair was removed to help achieve this.

In Victorian times (the 19th century), respectable women regarded natural beauty and sexual modesty highly. So returned a more modest fashion, without the masses of make up and elaborate hair-styles, and women were covered in clothes from head to toe.

In the 20th century we have experienced several different fashions. From the 1920s to the 1950s the sophisticated look was in, and the permed, blonde, body-hairless bombshell was fashionable. In the sixties the hippy revolution took the Western World by storm, and everyone, men, women and children, dressed and behaved as naturally as possible. Female body hair was left untouched and head hair was left long, loose and free. In fact, an interesting quote from this time comes from Lillian Roxon, a journalist commenting on the world of the young: 'In the seventies women will stop shaving their body hair. By 1975 every pretty girl will have hairy legs. Otherwise she will look old-fashioned.' She was too optimistic in her prediction; however, it cannot be denied that the passing of the hippy generation has left us with a more natural attitude towards body hair.

PUBIC HAIR

There are some interesting social changes regarding pubic hair throughout history. In 16th-century Europe it was removed, but by the 17th century it was fashionable to wear pubic wigs, called merkins (these are still available today in some sex shops). Representations of pubic hair in paintings reveals that before the 19th century the classic beauty lacked pubic hair, and it is only in paintings dating from the

Impressionist movement that glimpses of its existence can be found.

In this century, up to the mid-1940s, a woman's upper thigh and pubic region was only ever seen by her intimate friends; swimming costumes had little skirts or shorts attached to them, and the extension of what was considered the pubic region (down the thigh and up the abdomen) was accepted as normal. Only with the creation of the newer swimming costumes which allowed the upper thigh (and even more!) to be visible was the concept of the 'bikini line' invented. Before this time, no such demarcation of 'desired pubic hair' and 'undesired pubic hair' was made: it was all pubic hair and regarded in the same way. In its short life-time, the bikini line has changed shape and position depending upon the fashion of a particular summer, and each year women have had to remove a little bit more of their pubic hair so that they do not reveal any 'undesired pubic hair' while wearing their swimming costumes. It might make some women feel better to know that the 'high leg' fashion of swimming costumes since 1990 required almost 100 per cent of women to shape artificially their pubic region. At least in nudist beaches there is no such concept of a bikini line, and the natural pubic hair line is often admired.

EYEBROWS
These have also changed a lot through the ages. In the 17th and 18th centuries women plucked and shaved their eyebrows (and their hair line at the forehead) to give a surprised, naive look (this practice started initially as part of women's attempt to look chaste in the eyes of the Church, and only later became modified into a fashion). Later, false eyebrows were made, with such materials as mouse skin, and by the end of the 18th century eyebrows were either pencilled in or plucked. In the 20th century initially the nonexis-

tent eyebrow with only a thin pencil line in its place was fashionable, but more recently, with the advent of Brooke Shields and other fashion models, thick, natural eyebrows are considered attractive.

Non-sexual Attitudes towards Women's Body Hair

Above I have described the sexual and physical attitudes towards body hair in different Western cultures, and how body hair has been used by fashion, aesthetics, the Church and to establish sexual differentiation, all aiming to promote a particular 'look'. Sadly, at different times through history body hair has been used to symbolize other attitudes, and these have invariably been unfavourable towards the woman with body hair.

One horrific example is the witch hunts of the Counter-reformation of the 17th century, which were actually propagated by the State with the aim to obtain, by force, land and money from rich widows. These lonely ladies were singled out by the State, their names were slandered and they were accused of being witches. A belief that body hair in women was associated with the devil was used to take these women by force, shave them completely (in order to reveal 'satanic marks'), murder them and then take all their possessions.

Another awful symbol of body hair in women was the Victorian invention of freak shows. By displaying all the different 'freaks', the 'normal' people could go home feeling virtuous and clean. One of the freaks was the bearded woman, and she along with all the other anomalies of nature was treated like an animal by her keepers, and displayed to be pitied and ridiculed by the masses. Compare this attitude to that of the Duke of Alcala in 17th-century Spain, when he came across a bearded woman with a baby. She had had three miscarriages before she was 37 years old, and then she gradually developed facial hair before she at last gave birth at the age of 52. He had her portrait painted, and it showed a beautiful, albeit bearded woman, suckling her baby. He succeeded in showing her womanhood despite her abundant facial hair.

Tribal Attitudes towards Body Hair

Looking at different tribes throughout the world reveals that they too have dealt with body hair in various ways. Either removal of body hair is part of ritualistic behaviour, or body hair is regarded as aesthetically unpleasing and better removed. There is not that much sexual differentiation regarding attitudes towards body hair, and more often than not, both men and women remove it. Let me give you some examples:

Apparently the Brazilian Indians (men and women) have sparse body hair, and what they have is plucked out because they consider it to be ugly. This includes their eyebrows and eyelashes as well as all body hair, so that only the hair on their heads is left (this to protect them from the sun).

In the South Pacific Islands some tribes remove all underarm hair (in men and women), but many admire pubic hair in women, and the pubic hair of virgins is combed and oiled with care.

In Central Africa the Bakitara people use body hair as part of ritualistic behaviour; young girls approaching marriage have all their body hair shaved except for their pubic hair, which is plucked out by their mothers over a three-day period.

In Zambia a certain tribe have all their young adults (boys and girls) remove, by plucking, their newly-growing pubic and underarm hair.

References

W. Cooper, Hair: Sex, Society, Symbolism, New York: Stein and Day Publishers, 1971.

R. B. Greenblatt, V. B. Mahesh, R. D. Gabrell (eds.), *The Cause and Management of Hirsutism*, Parthenon Publishing, 1987.

2

HOW HAIR GROWS

Introduction

It might appear that men and women only have hair in certain areas of their bodies, however this is not so. Except for a few small areas (the lips, soles of the feet, palms of the hands and parts of the genitals) we are covered with hair; the reason you cannot see it in some areas is because the hairs there are absolutely tiny. All hairs protrude from small openings in the skin called *pores*, underneath which are hair *follicles*, from which each hair grows. From birth the number of follicles we have on our bodies is fixed, and men and women have the same number. What changes as we get older is the quality of the hair that grows from these follicles – in most cases hair changes to become thicker and longer. Most women believe that they have too many of these thicker hairs over their bodies, and some actually seek medical advice for reassurances about their femininity. The majority of women who have a lot of body hair are completely normal. Only a tiny minority of women have an underlying illness that causes excess body hair; these illnesses of course need to be investigated and treated.

Types of Hair

The hair on our bodies ranges from being tiny, blond, straight and fine to long, black, thick and curly. Between these two extremes lie all different varieties, and if you look at your own body you should find at least several different types of hair.

Doctors, instead of considering hair as a continuous spectrum encompassing all physical varieties, have classified it into several different types, each having different characteristics. These characteristics are related either to how the hair looks, or to how the hair behaves under different body conditions (i.e. the ways it changes its physical appearance and the dynamics of its growth). This will be made clearer to you as you read further.

Regarding the physical appearance of hair, it has been classified into the following two types:

1. Vellus hair
   These are the tiny, blond, fine hairs. A baby's body is covered with these hairs at birth, and you might be able to see them on your own body if you look at your inner lower arm. They are practically invisible, and are described as being less than 2 mm long, with very little colour to them and made up of only one kind of hair material (described later).

2. Terminal hair
   This type of hair includes all the other physical varieties that are found on our bodies. For example, the hair on your head, under your arms, on your legs, etc. This hair is made of two materials, is longer than 2 mm and has a range of different colours from blond to black. Its thickness varies from very fine to coarse, its shape from straight to fuzzy.

As I have mentioned, hair can change under different conditions of the body, and these conditions are almost inevitably related to the body's hormonal state. Hair can change in two ways:

1. The hair can change from the type it was at birth (vellus or terminal) to the other hair type, but it cannot change back. For example, vellus hair over the lower legs of a baby changes to terminal hair during puberty, or terminal hair over the head of a baby changes to vellus hair when that baby grows to be an older, balding man. Neither of these changes will ever be reversed (under the normal conditions of life).

2. The physical characteristics of a terminal hair can change under different hormonal conditions throughout our lives, and for each hair can change more than once. So, for example, a fairly fine terminal hair in a bikini line after puberty can change to a thicker more pubic-like hair later on in life, or a thick hair in the lower abdominal mid-line can change to a finer one during pregnancy, only to change back again once the pregnancy is over. It is important to understand that any change to the thickness and length of a hair will be coupled with a corresponding change to the size and depth of the hair follicle (described in detail later).

Next, by looking at the behaviour of different areas of hair under different hormonal conditions, two further categories have been defined, and whether a hair falls into one category or the other depends upon where it is situated on the body, as follows:

1. **Asexual hair**   The areas of *asexual hair* are: the eyebrows, lashes and the hair on our heads[1].
   These areas of hair are of the terminal hair type at birth, and are not under the control of what are called the sex hormones (see below). Thus what difference there is in these hairs between males and females is not related to the levels of these hormones, but is determined by other factors.

2. **Sexual hair**   These areas of hair are vellus at birth, and under the influence of *sex hormones* they turn into terminal hairs.

Let me explain what is meant by the sex hormones: men and women differ in many ways, and one of these is in the amounts and kinds of hormones each sex produces. Women produce a large amount of the female sex hormones, called *oestrogens*, and only a small amount of the male sex hormones, called *androgens* (an example of an androgen that most people have heard of is *testosterone*, and this is in fact the main androgen produced in our bodies). Men do the reverse: they produce a large amount of testosterone and a small amount of oestrogens. The exact amounts of each hormone that men and women produce differs in different people, but there is a range that is regarded as normal (just as there is a range for each of the other hormones in our body that is regarded as normal), and men have about ten times as much testosterone in their bodies as women. These hormones circulate in our bodies and enter different tissues (for example, skin, fat, muscle) and produce an effect in that tissue (for example, when testosterone enters muscles, it makes them increase in bulk).

---

[1]Usually scalp hair is included in the category of asexual hair, however there is a hormonal basis to one pattern of balding, i.e. balding at the temples. Usually it is seen in men, but women with excessive amounts of the male hormones can also develop this balding pattern. Scalp hair therefore is not completely of the asexual kind.

When these two sex hormones enter skin and hair tissue they have different effects on the growth and quality of sexual hairs: testosterone makes the hair longer, coarser and faster-growing, whereas oestrogens slow down its growth and make it finer. However, the effects of testosterone on the hair by far dominates the effects of the oestrogens, in both men and women. This means that an area of sexual hair in contact with a high level of testosterone will gradually change from being very fine and short to very coarse and long (regardless of the level of oestrogens), but the same area of hair in contact with a lower level of testosterone will develop into being less coarse and not quite as long. Thus, if an area of sexual hair is in contact with one level of testosterone for some time and the level then changes, the characteristics (thickness, length and rate of growth) of that hair will change accordingly. These characteristics of sexual hair can change many times in any one area according to the level of testosterone.

Where are these areas of sexual hair? They are:

• the pubic and underarm region,
• the legs and arms,
• the face, chest and abdomen, and
• the back and shoulders.

However, one important way in which these sexual areas differ from each other is in their sensitivity to testosterone. Some areas, the pubic and underarm regions, need only very low levels of testosterone (as found in women) to change the hair from being fine to coarse, and as a result both men and women have coarse hair in these areas. Other areas of sexual hair need very high levels of testosterone to change the quality of the hair (e.g. the back and shoulders), and so only those few men with very high levels of testosterone have thick hair in these areas. All the other areas fall somewhere in between.

Can we see other examples of this on our bodies? The clearest example is the hair over the face of a man compared with that of a woman: all men have testosterone levels high enough to change the hairs here to coarse and fast-growing ones, whereas in a woman they are usually fine and short. Compare this to chest hairs, which are coarse in only a relatively small proportion of men. Lastly, comparing the thighs of men and women you will find that almost all men and about half the women have terminal hair here, although in an average man this terminal hair is a bit longer and thicker than that of an average woman.

The above discussion should have convinced you that, to a large extent, it is the level of testosterone in your body that determines where you will be hairy and how hairy you will be in each area. Also, it should be clear that there is no such thing as a particularly 'male' or 'female' pattern of hair growth. There is only one pattern of hair growth, and this pattern is the one that is seen as you increase the level of testosterone. Since men and women both have testosterone in them, they have the same pattern of hair growth. What is different is the extent to which that pattern is expressed: men tend to express more hair because they have more testosterone, while women tend to express less hair. There is no cut-off point above which one can say 'this is a male distribution of hair' and below which one can say 'this is a female distribution', rather there is a lot of overlap in the middle and there are two extremes, the hairy extreme where men tend to fall, and the hair-free extreme where women tend to fall.

The Structure, Growth Cycle and Transformation of Hair and Follicle

Let me now spend some time discussing the hair and its follicle, and describe how they both grow and change in cycles.

THE STRUCTURE OF HAIR AND FOLLICLE

The upper layer of skin dips downwards every few millimetres to form tube-like structures called follicles, and from each of these follicles protrudes a hair (sometimes more than one). These follicles are continuous with the skin, and are therefore constant structures which remain intact even after a hair is pulled out.

Into the upper part of each follicle a gland, called the *sebaceous gland*, secretes an oily substance called *sebum*. The opening of the follicle at the surface of the skin is called the pore, and this, like the follicle, is a constant structure. The hair, its follicle and the one or more sebaceous glands attached to the follicle is called the *pilosebaceous unit* (see Figure 1). As a general rule, the thicker and longer a hair is, the bigger and deeper its follicle.

Sebaceous glands are part of the hair follicle, but the size of these glands differs greatly in different areas. For example, over the scalp, forehead, upper cheeks and nose they are very large, whereas over the arms and neck they are small. Their size increases under the influence of testosterone, and the bigger they are, the more sebum they release. The main function of sebum is to lubricate and prevent water loss from both skin and hair. (During puberty the sebaceous glands become very active, mainly stimulated by the increase in testosterone, and often release too much sebum, which plays a part in the development of blackheads, pimples and acne).

The hair consists of three parts: the hair *shaft*, which protrudes above the skin, the hair *root*, which is below the skin, and the hair *bulb*, which is the thickened part of the root deepest in the skin. At the very depth of the hair bulb, in an area called the *dermal papilla*, is a group of cells called the *germinating cells* (see Figure 2), and it is believed that all hair growth begins from these cells.

The hair root is surrounded by the hair follicle, which

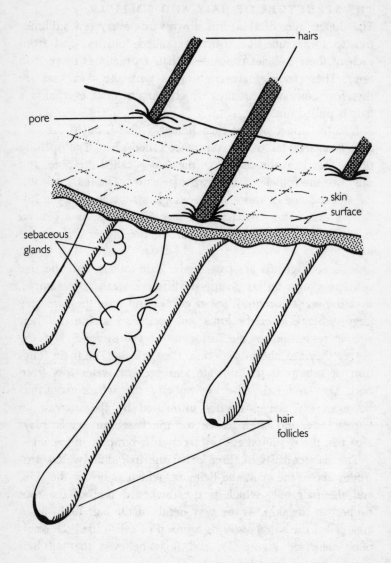

Figure 1: The pilosebaceous unit

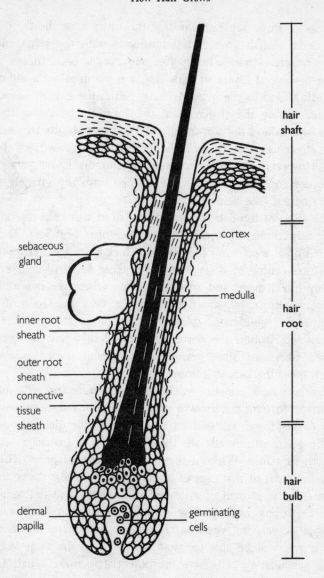

Figure 2: The structure of hair and follicle

consists of three separate sheaths: the inner root sheath, the outer root sheath (which is continuous with the skin) and the connective tissue sheath (see Figure 2). Each sheath is made of several layers of cells that are involved with either providing food to the growing hair, giving the hair its shape, or maintaining the structure of the follicle. The connective tissue sheath and the upper part of the outer sheath are constant structures that do not change with the growth of the hair. However, the inner root sheath and the lower part of the outer root sheath grow and change with the growth of the hair itself (see below).

The shaft of the hair is made up of dead hair cells that are compactly cemented together into the form of fibres. Each cell is full of a protein called keratin. Thick hairs are constructed with a central medulla, which has these keratin-filled cells loosely interwoven, and an outer cortex where the hair cells are very compactly woven together. In very fine hairs, for example the vellus hairs, there is no medulla.

Scattered around the cortex embedded between the keratinized fibres are little granules of pigment, called melanin, which gives the hair its colour.

The hair bulb contains within it many different cells that are involved with the growth of the hair, but I shall describe only two of them, the germinating cells and the melanocytes.

The germinating cells are those cells that are crucial to the growth of a hair. Without them the hair cannot grow. They are equivalent to that part of a flowering bulb that starts and maintains the growth of a flower; if you prise out the centre of a flowering bulb you will have destroyed its ability to grow a flower, but you can chop off other bits of the bulb and it will still be able to grow a flower. In the same way, these germinating cells have the potential to make a hair (as well as the inner sheath and the lower part of the outer sheath of the follicle); from the beginning to the end of the growth of a hair these cells divide continually, and the new cells that are made slowly push their way up the hair follicle, either to cement themselves together to make the hair root or to migrate to the sides to make the inner sheath. As the hair continues to grow, what was the hair root initially becomes the hair shaft.

The melanocytes are also situated in the hair bulb, but closer to its upper end. These cells produce a pigment called melanin which is released as granules which get taken up into the growing hair and become scattered throughout the cortex of the hair. This melanin gives hair its colour, and the more melanin there is within a hair shaft the darker the hair will be. Thus, blond hairs have very little of this pigment in them and black hairs have a lot. For a fuller discussion, see page 54.

THE GROWTH CYCLE OF A FOLLICLE AND ITS HAIR

Now that you understand the basic ingredients that make up a follicle and its hair, we can go on to discuss how they grow.

Throughout a person's life span each hair follicle under-goes repeated growth cycles, so that any one follicle may have produced and shed between 10 and 400 hairs.

Briefly, the growth cycle of the follicle is made up of two long phases and one short, intermediate phase. The first phase of the cycle is the *growth phase*. This starts when the follicle begins to grow a hair from the germinating cells and ends when a full-length hair is produced. After a brief inter-mediate period (the *involution phase* – see below) the second major phase of the cycle begins: this is the *resting phase*. This begins when the hair has reached its full length and ends when a new hair begins a new growth cycle underneath. The *involution phase* is the transition of a hair root, bulb and follicle from growing to resting (see Figure 3).

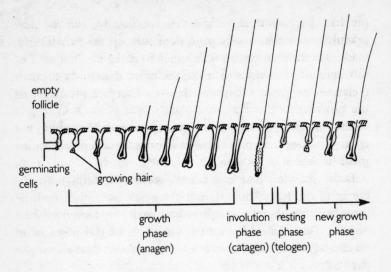

empty
follicle

germinating
cells

growing hair

growth
phase
(anagen)

involution
phase
(catagen)

resting
phase
(telogen)

new growth
phase

Figure 3: Growth cycle of a hair follicle

In any area of hair all the follicles are at different stages of
the growth cycle: some are newly growing, some are just at
the end of the growth phase, and others are in different
stages of the resting phase. You can compare this to those
animals who have synchronized hair growth, where all the
hairs are in the same phase of growth and the cycle ends
with a seasonal moult (for example cats or dogs). A whole
area of hair can all be stimulated into entering the growth
phase together by pulling them all out by the roots (for
example, when you wax your legs).

Let me discuss these phases in more detail.

The Growth Phase (Anagen)

During this phase the germinating cells first of all start making the hair bulb; this slowly grows until the size of the bulb
is about one third that of the hair follicle. As new cells are
added to the bulb its upper end starts to become the shaft of

the hair root. Into this shaft the melanocytes release their granules of melanin pigment. Gradually, as more cells are made, the hair eventually reaches the top of the follicle (by this time it is lubricated with sebum and pigmented with melanin) and begins to protrude out of the skin and continues growing in this way until the growth phase is over (see Figure 3). The tip of a newly growing hair is very fine, and as it gets longer it gradually gets thicker until it reaches its usual thickness.

Each hair has a fixed length of time during which it is in the growing phase, and for each area of hair this length of time is different. For example, the follicles on the head continue growing a hair for between three and eight years, those on the thighs for between four and six months, and those on the fingers for a few weeks. If you cut a hair which is in the middle of its growth phase it will not grow for longer than its fixed time. What happens is that it continues to grow until it reaches the end of its growth phase and then stops growing, so that its final length will be shorter than that of the adjacent hair which was not cut.

You can recognize a hair in the growth phase by the way the root looks when it is plucked (see Figure 4). The root is long and white and at the bottom there is often a little black spot. The long white root is in fact the inner sheath of the follicle and the hair bulb. If you regularly pluck your eyebrows you can see this root in the newly-growing hairs.

How many hairs in a particular area are in the growth phase? The numbers differ for the different areas: over the face it is believed that only 20 to 30 per cent of the hairs are in the growth phase, and over the legs even less. In the scalp the majority of hairs are growing.

The Involution Phase (Catagen)
When the growth phase has finished, the hair bulb, root and

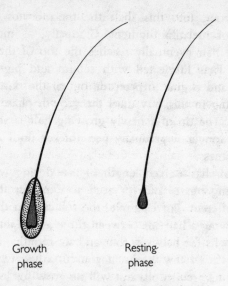

Growth   Resting
phase   phase

Figure 4: *Hair bulb and hair in different phases of the growth cycle*

follicle change their structure before they enter the resting phase. The transition between the growing phase and the resting phase is called the involution phase.

The first change is in the melanocytes, which stop producing pigment; the next is in the bulb, which stops producing new cells. The long bulb (and surrounding follicle) then somehow get absorbed into the surrounding tissues, and the germinating cells, because they have migrated downwards and the lower third of the follicle has been absorbed, end up *below the bottom of the follicle*. The end of the hair, instead of having a long bulb, develops a 'club bulb' which becomes firmly attached to the base of the shallow follicle (this 'club bulb' and follicle is about one third of the length of a bulb and follicle in the growing phase – see Figure 3). To understand the later discussion of electrolysis it is important to visualize this properly; the germinating cells, which are those that are essential to the growth of the next hair, are embedded in skin tissue *below* the end of the follicle.

The Resting Phase (Telogen)

The follicle and hair in the resting phase remains as it is, with its 'club bulb', until the resting phase is over. Just as there are specific lengths of time for a follicle to grow, so there are specific lengths of time for a follicle to rest, and different areas of hair have different resting times – weeks for thigh hair, months for hair on the scalp. As the end of the follicle's resting phase approaches, the germinating cells underneath start growing and organizing another growing bulb and hair (i.e. it is the beginning of a new growth phase). This new hair will grow alongside the old hair, thus loosening the latter's attachments and making it either fall out naturally or be pulled out easily with brushing, washing, etc. You can recognize hairs in the resting phase (take a look at your hairbrush) by their short unpigmented 'club' ends (in fact you should only see this type of root in your brush). How many hairs in different areas are in the resting phase? Over the face about 30 to 50 per cent of the hairs are resting, and over the legs up to 70 to 80 per cent are resting.

Dormant Hair Follicles

There is one other state that a hair follicle can be in, and this is the *dormant* state. These follicles are effectively 'hibernating' until something triggers them into action. They have no hair coming out of them, and the follicle is an empty tube. At any given time about 20 per cent of our hair follicles are in the dormant phase.

TRANSFORMATION OF HAIR AND FOLLICLE

Is there a reason why follicles and hair should go through many cycles like this? Why do they not behave like the nails on our hands, continuing to grow and grow? The reason is probably that as a result of this system of repeated cycles the follicle has the ability to change its size and depth in a step-wise manner according to the level of testosterone in our bodies. In this way the follicle can not only increase its size (and thus also the thickness of the hair) and increase its depth (and thus the length of the hair) with higher testosterone levels but can also *decrease its size with lower levels of testosterone*.

Earlier I described how testosterone can affect the thickness, rate of growth and length of a hair, and I mentioned that the size and the depth of the follicle change accordingly. When does all this happen?

Each time a hair begins a new growth phase, depending upon the level of testosterone around at the time the follicle can change its size just a little bit. And each time the hair goes through a new cycle, the size can change a little more, so that after a few cycles what was a rather small follicle, producing a rather fine hair, has become in the presence of higher levels of testosterone a large follicle producing a thick, faster-growing hair. This is how those tiny vellus hairs around the chin of a boy gradually become the thick terminal beard hairs of a man: a gradual increase in the testosterone level producing a step-by-step increase in the size and depth of the follicle at the beginning of each growth cycle. Likewise, a woman with fine hair on her face gradually develops thicker and thicker hair in the presence of high testosterone.

The same transformation can occur in all other areas of sexual hair. It is important to remember that the reverse can occur also: if a woman has high testosterone levels and develops thick hair, then when this testosterone level is reduced to normal, the hairs and follicles will slowly become smaller and finer until they are the finest and slowest-growing kind of terminal hair (but remember, they can never revert to vellus hair again).

The Pattern of Women's Hair Growth

By now you should have some idea of how hair grows, what determines its thickness and length, and why we get hairier. There is a pattern of hair growth through life that the average woman will follow, and studies of hair growth in different areas in women have revealed how common body hair actually is.

HAIR GROWTH DURING A WOMAN'S LIFETIME
At birth a baby (boy or girl) is covered in vellus hair, except for the terminal hair over his or her asexual areas (head, eyelashes and eyebrows) and those areas that are devoid of hair throughout life (lips, palms of hands, soles of feet and genitals).

From birth a hormone called *growth hormone* is released from the brain which is essential for the growth of the child and also causes a small increase in hair growth over the limb extremities.

From around age 8 a gland called the *adrenal gland* increases its activity and produces small levels of androgen. In girls this is believed to be what stimulates the onset of breast budding and the beginning of pubic hair production, as well as causing an increase in the amount of hair growth over the limbs.

Around puberty the ovaries become activated and they produce oestrogens and testosterone. From here, secondary sexual characteristics continue to develop (breast development, pubic and underarm hair, maturation of the genital tract and the development of the female contours), menstruation begins and limbs continue to grow more hair.

As a woman passes puberty and enters womanhood the level of testosterone remains constant, however her body continues to get hairier: the extension of the pubic triangle, moustache, leg hair, abdominal hair, etc. This is thought to occur because the hair follicles are not only sensitive to the level of testosterone but also to how long the testosterone has been present, i.e. somehow the follicles get more sensitive to the presence of testosterone with time.

With the onset of the menopause the ovaries stop working and thus stop producing their oestrogens and testosterone. At about the same time the androgen glands begin to reduce their testosterone output. The net effect is a reduction of testosterone and a cessation of oestrogens. This causes the hair follicles over the trunk slowly to reduce in size until they eventually stop growing any hairs at all. For some reason (which remains unclear) facial hairs continue to increase in number, and tend to be thick and coarse, especially over the chin, edges of the upper lip and cheeks.

PREVALENCE OF HAIR GROWTH IN DIFFERENT PARTS OF A WOMAN'S BODY

Two studies have been carried out on women (one study looked at only white British women, the other study did not specify nationality, race or colour) to find out the prevalence of hairs in different areas of the body at different ages. The results show clearly that women are naturally more hairy than we are lead to believe:

- Facial hair
  About 25 per cent of young women have noticeable hair on the face, in 10 per cent it is easily seen. The most common area is above the upper lip. Up to the menopause facial hair does not increase that much, but afterwards there is a gradual increase for the rest of a

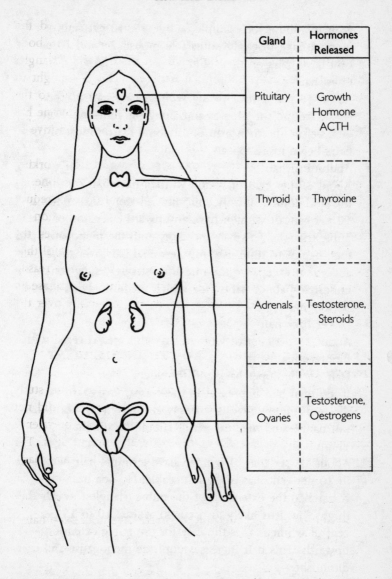

Gland	Hormones Released
Pituitary	Growth Hormone ACTH
Thyroid	Thyroxine
Adrenals	Testosterone, Steroids
Ovaries	Testosterone, Oestrogens

Figure 5: The glands in a woman's body that can, when not functioning properly, cause excess body hair

woman's life – for example, at age 65, 40 per cent of
women have an easily noticeable moustache and 10 per
cent have hairs on their chin.

- Chest hair
  About 15 per cent of young women have hair on their
  chest, around the nipples and along the mid-line. Even
  well before the menopause, for some reason most of these
  hairs begin to disappear.

- Abdominal hair
  About 30 per cent of young women have hair on their
  lower abdomen, mostly concentrated along the mid-line.
  10 per cent of women have an upward extension of their
  pubic triangle. This hair increases until the menopause and
  then begins to diminish. Any terminal hair over the upper
  abdomen, except for the mid-line, strongly suggests an
  underlying abnormality, for which medical advice should
  be sought.

- Lower back hair
  About 15 per cent of women have this area covered with
  fine terminal hair.

- Hair on the upper back and shoulders
  If terminal hair is present in these areas anywhere except
  the mid-line it suggests strongly an underlying hormonal
  imbalance, and medical advice should be sought.

- Thigh hair
  About 40 per cent of women have terminal hair here, and
  in 20 per cent it is easily noticeable. No one has
  researched the extension of the pubic triangle towards the
  thighs, but it is likely to occur in at least 10 to 15 per
  cent of women, as is the case for the pubic extension
  upwards. This hair increases until the menopause and then
  diminishes.

- Lower leg hair
  Almost all young women have noticeable hair here, and it

increases as we get older until the menopause and then goes.

The Regulation of Women's Hair Growth

Above I gave you the results of two studies that reveal how common body hair is in the female population. It cannot be possible that all these women have testosterone levels that are above the average range. There must be other factors in our bodies that determine how hairy we are, other factors that affect the growth of body hair, that help to convert that fine, downy vellus hair to coarser, darker terminal hair. What are they?

There are in fact four main components to the interaction between the hair follicle and testosterone, and each of these components plays a part in determining how hairy you will be and where you will be hairy. Their net effect is what you see over your body. These components are as follows.

LEVELS OF TESTOSTERONE

Testosterone comes from three sources: the ovaries (25 per cent of the total), the adrenal glands (25 per cent) and the conversion of pre-testosterone to testosterone in skin cells (50 per cent). I have already described that the higher the levels of testosterone in your body, the hairier you will be. If from any of these three sources too much testosterone is made, you will have levels at the higher end of average (or even higher) and you will tend to be hairier than average.

LEVELS OF 'FREE TESTOSTERONE'

Testosterone, which is present in the body as tiny molecules, circulates in the blood and produces its effect on the hair follicles by entering the cells of the follicles and somehow activating hair growth. The testosterone circulates in the body in two forms; in one form it is bound onto a larger molecule[2] which makes the testosterone too big to enter into the follicle cells – thus in this bound form it is inactive.

The other form is unbound, or 'free testosterone', and in this form it is free to enter the cells and have its effect. About 99 per cent of the testosterone is in the bound, inactive form, and only 1 per cent is in the 'free' form. If you happen to have a higher level of 'free testosterone', despite normal levels of total testosterone, it would be likely to stimulate more hair growth. A higher level of 'free testosterone' occurs when the body makes a reduced amount of testosterone-binding molecules.

CONVERSION OF 'FREE TESTOSTERONE' TO 'HAIR-PROMOTING' ANDROGEN

The main androgen in the body is testosterone. The unbound, free testosterone enters hair follicle cells and is converted (with the help of an enzyme called 5α reductase) into another androgen, called dihydrotestosterone. It is this androgen, in the hair follicle cells, that actually stimulates the hair follicle to grow a terminal hair, and to grow a thicker terminal hair if there is a large amount of dihydrotestosterone around. If your body had a really high level of testosterone in it but was unable to convert any of it to dihydrotestosterone in the follicle cells, your skin would be almost as smooth as a baby's bottom! We all convert roughly the same amount of testosterone to dihydrotestosterone, however those of us who convert a little more, will be that little bit more hairy.

THE SENSITIVITY OF THE HAIR FOLLICLE TO TESTOSTERONE

I have already mentioned that different areas of (sexual) hair

---

[2] Either sex hormone binding globulin (SHBG), or albumin.

are sensitive to different levels of testosterone; the more sensitive an area is, the hairier it will become when in contact with testosterone. We all have roughly the same sensitivities in some regions, so that all of us get very hairy under the arm and in the pubic region. However, some women are more sensitive than others, and those women who are more sensitive will tend to grow more hair in more areas even though they have the same level of testosterone in their bodies as have those that are less sensitive.

What determines how big a role each of the above four components will play in your body? Why is it that some women have so little body hair because of an 'underplay' of these components while other women have too much body hair because of an 'overplay' of these components?

How the above four factors interplay is just a small part of the enormous developmental process that goes in our bodies throughout our lives and which determines almost all of our physical characteristics. The main factors which influence this development are:

1. Race
   Distribution and quality of hair for the different races is as characteristic as skin colour. The Mongolian race (including the Chinese, Japanese, Koreans, American Indians and Inuit/Eskimos) have less body and facial hair (which is also less coarse and sparser) than have Caucasians. And of the Caucasians, hair growth is heavier in those of Mediterranean descent than in those of Nordic descent. In fact, Mongolians actually have a smaller number of hair follicles than have Caucasians, which means that a hairy Mongolian can have hair as coarse as that of a Caucasian, but it will always be sparser. More interesting is that Japanese men and women have similar levels of testosterone in their bodies as have Caucasian

men and women, but if high levels of testosterone are given to Japanese women they do not become hairy, whereas similar levels given to Caucasian women would induce a marked increase in body hair. This shows that there is a large variation in the way that the hair follicles of different races respond to testosterone.

2. Inherited characteristics

Just as you inherited the size of your nose, or your height, or the colour of your eyes from your parents, so you inherited the hairiness of your body from them (from either your father or mother). In fact you even inherit the pattern of hairiness from them. We can take the inheritance one step further and say, if your mother had a lot of body hair because she converted too much testosterone to dihydrotestosterone, then if you are hairy it is likely to be for the same reason.

3. Other factors

There are a few minor factors that also influence hair growth, although these play a very small role in comparison to the two mentioned above.

a. I have mentioned the growth hormone: this increases the rate and thickness of hair.

b. Any increase in skin temperature will also tend to increase hair growth. This is thought to be due to increased blood flow to the follicle, which enables more nutrients to reach the follicle and allows it to grow bigger. For example, in the summer months our bodies tend to get hairier; similarly, when a part of the body is in a plaster cast for some time, the hairs underneath become longer and thicker.

c. During pregnancy the body's hormones change drastically. Usually body hair is reduced during this time, but sometimes women complain of a slight increase in hair. Both are normal physiological states.

d. In one study doctors found that after an unsuccessful love affair women would become temporarily more hairy; this is due to a temporary increase in testosterone.

e. Some clinicians have postulated that stress (physical and psychological) might lead to an increase in body hair by increasing testosterone released by the stress glands, i.e. the adrenal glands.

f. For some reason women in psychiatric hospitals tend to be hairier than average. The reason for this is unclear. Could it be the lack of razors?

Medical Definitions of Excess Body Hair

There is a medical term for women (and children) who develop 'excessive' hair growth, in distributions usually seen only in men. It is called hirsutism; and a woman is said to be hirsute. What is normally meant by the 'male distribution' of hair is: on the abdomen, chest, face, shoulders and back. However, the distinction is not completely clear since, as I have described, hair distribution and growth in men and women is all part of one spectrum, with men tending to fall at the hairier end and women at the hairless end. There is no 'natural female distribution' or 'natural male distribution', each one being completely distinct and having its own limitations.

If you asked a number of doctors to describe the difference between normal hair distribution and hirsute hair distribution you would probably meet with blank faces, and certainly with different answers. There is no fixed cut-off point below which a woman is 'normal' and above which a woman is 'hirsute'. For example, a Mediterranean woman with hair over her thighs would be regarded by her neighbours as normal, whereas a Japanese woman with the same distribution would probably be regarded as hirsute. Lots of such factors have to be taken into account when deciding if a female is hirsute or not. Much more often than not it is the woman herself who has fixed, preconceived ideas about what is 'normal female hair distribution', and this because she has been brainwashed by society. It is true however that any woman with hair over her upper back and shoulders, upper abdomen and (markedly so) on her face almost invariably has an underlying hormonal problem and should seek medical advice.

The medical term for another kind of excess body hair, which is far less common, is *hypertrichosis*. This is seen in children, females and males, and describes excessive hair growth over the entire body surface regardless of whether the area is a 'masculine' one or not. The hair itself is not thickened as it is in hirsutism, but is usually fine, and longer than normal. Certain drugs and underlying chronic illnesses can lead to hypertrichosis (these are mentioned below).

Seeking Medical Help for Excess Body Hair

It is a common belief held by women that they have too much body hair. It should not surprise anyone that women hold this belief, when all around them there is 'evidence' that female body hair is abnormal: pictures of hairless models and actresses in magazines, posters and films, male partners expecting women to have totally smooth bodies, and advertisements for hair removal products talking about 'disfiguring', 'unsightly' or 'unacceptable' hair growth that should be removed in order to restore 'femininity'. No wonder GPs and hospital doctors see thousands of women each year with worries about excess body hair. Men would also arrive in droves if women started expecting them always to have a full chest of hair, if all male models and actors had hairy chests, and if advertisements existed for products that grew chest hair and spoke of 'the disfiguringly smooth chest' or 'the unsightly bare chest' or 'unacceptably hairless chest'. If only...

Women approach doctors either because they are anxious about how unfeminine they are (because of their body hair) or because they really are worried about some underlying abnormality. Anxiety can range from mild worry and embarrassment to marked personality changes; feelings of persecution, neurotic preoccupation with body hair, withdrawal from sexual relationships and even society. The kind of worries women have are, for example, fear of turning into a man, or fear of some dreadful illness. Yet of all the women that reach a doctor 99 per cent have nothing wrong with them. Only 1 per cent have an underlying illness which has to be dealt with. The other 99 per cent are women with inherited or racial characteristics that have made them relatively hairy by an 'overplay' of one or more of the components of the testosterone/hair follicle mechanism discussed earlier.

The doctor's task is not easy. Firstly, the 1 per cent with an underlying problem have to be identified and treated. Next the doctor has to convince the other 99 per cent that they are normal, despite the fact that most of society is telling them they are not. Lastly, the doctor is expected to prescribe something for these 99 per cent of women that will remove their body hair (and in fact some drugs do exist, see page 47).

How is it all done? The doctor first of all asks questions, then he or she examines the woman, and lastly he or she may (or may not) organize certain tests. Below is a description of the kind of consultation you can expect.

THE QUESTIONS ASKED

Family Background

The doctor must first find out about your family and ethnic history. Were your parents hairy? Did your mother have any problems with menstruation or conceiving? What are your ethnic roots? Are your sisters (if you have any) hairy? etc.

Pattern of Hair Growth

A knowledge of when the problem started and how quickly it progressed is very important; a gradual increase in body hair since puberty is usually normal, post-menopausal facial hair is also normal, but any rapid increase (over just a few months or a year) in body hair at any age, or the onset of sexual hair before puberty, is usually abnormal and will need further investigations.

The doctor will also want to ascertain the distribution and quality of your body hair: any hair over your upper back, shoulders, upper abdomen (but not at the mid-line), chest (but not mid-line or on the nipples) is abnormal, and always needs investigating. In women before the menopause thick hairs over the neck and cheeks is abnormal and also need investigating. Excess growth of fine hair all over the body may suggest another kind of illness (for example, anorexia nervosa).

Previous Medical History

Past and present illnesses are important; when the body is debilitated it can grow body hair in order to keep itself warm. Illnesses such as anorexia nervosa and malnutrition cause this kind of hair growth.

Questions about your menstrual cycle and fertility will give the doctor an idea of your hormone balance: when your periods started (if you are a young woman), how heavy and frequent they are, whether they are regular. If your menstrual cycle is normal it is unlikely that you have any underlying problem. The doctor will also need to know whether you have ever been pregnant, have had any miscarriages or have ever given birth. If there is evidence that you are ovulating (gained from a temperature chart or blood tests), or if you have ever been pregnant, it is almost inevitable that you are normal. If however, your periods are irregular and you have a problem with fertility then it is possible that there is an underlying problem, and you will be investigated further.

Questions about acne and obesity are important: the presence of acne (at times other than puberty) suggests a hormonal imbalance, and obesity can either cause an imbalance of hormones or can be the result of an imbalance.

Hormonal Imbalances and Virilization

The imbalance of certain other body hormones can produce excess body hair. In adults these are the growth hormone and cortisol. Symptoms caused by these hormones when in excess include: weight gain, muscle weakness, purple stretch marks, a deep, coarse voice, coarsening of the features, and enlargement of the hands and feet. In children a decrease in the thyroid hormone can lead to the growth of fine, long hair over the whole body.

The doctor must exclude the possibility of virilization (this is the pattern of changes that occur in the body when there has been a sharp rise in testosterone over weeks or months) which is always abnormal. Symptoms may include: deepening of the voice, sudden increase in hairiness, increased libido, reduced breast tissue, increased muscle mass, disruption of menstrual cycle and balding over the temples.

Drug History

Certain drugs cause an increase in body hair. Most of these drugs can be substituted for another type if unwanted hair growth occurs. In some of these drugs the effect is reversible, but in others it is only partially reversible. These drugs can be divided into two groups according to the pattern of hair growth and the underlying mechanism:

1. The androgenic drugs

These basically have the same effect as testosterone, and
increase body hair in the sexual areas; usually beard and
moustache hair first, then on the chest, nipples, abdomen
and lastly the back. The hair that grows is usually coarse,
terminal hair. Most of these drugs (at the usual doses) only
cause an increase in body hair in those women that are
already hairier than average, i.e. those women who have an
'overplay' of the interaction between testosterone and hair
follicle. On stopping the drug, although the hair growth
diminishes within months, some body hair may not return
to its pre-treatment level (if a conversion of vellus to
terminal hair has occurred). So the general rule is to avoid
being given these androgenic drugs if you are already
hairier than average. The following is a list of such drugs:

a. Certain oral contraceptives

There is some suggestion that certain oral contraceptives,
especially in the past, have led to increased body hair. I
could not find any evidence to support this claim, but
this does not mean that a link does not exist.
Theoretically, certain oral contraceptives with a
predominance of male hormone could increase body
hair, but this has not been documented as far as I can
tell. And there are plenty of oral contraceptives with no
male hormone effects (see page 48).

b. Testosterone

In sufficient quantities testosterone will almost always
cause an increase in body hair in women, and may go
on to produce other virilizing effects. Testosterone is
sometimes given to women for the treatment of breast
cancer and aplastic anaemias, and low doses are used
with oestrogens in hormone replacement therapy (HRT).

c. Danazol

This drug is a weak androgen (i.e. a weak male

hormone), and is used in the treatment of endometriosis, cystic breast conditions and angioneurotic oedema. It causes an increase in body hair in about 5 per cent of women when given at the higher dose of 800 mg/day. This is reversible in some women when the drug is stopped, but others continue to have the increased body hair.

d. Cortisone and prednisolone
High doses of these steroids, given over long periods of time, have been known to increase body hair. The effect is reversible.

e. Cyclosporin
This is an immunosuppressant drug used in transplant patients. Sometimes hair growth is a side-effect, and it is not completely reversible.

f. Anabolic steroids
These are used by women for improvement of athletic performance. Some of these behave like testosterone, and have caused increased body hair in a proportion of women.

2. The nonhormonal drugs
These produce a different pattern of hair growth, called hypertrichosis. The hair is always finer terminal hair rather than coarse, and new growth appears over the temples, forehead, abdomen and back, while increased growth may occur over the back of the arms and over the legs. This kind of hair growth is most often seen in children (the underarm and pubic regions are spared), and can be prevented if careful monitoring and timely action is taken. In most cases, hair growth caused by these drugs is reversible within a few months of stopping medication. The drugs are:

a. Phenytoin
This drug is used for controlling epilepsy, and is most

commonly associated with hypertrichosis. Increased hair occurs in about 5 to 10 per cent of patients, and the most commonly affected areas are the limbs (and sometimes a moustache develops or hair grows on the trunk). Hair growth occurs within two to three months of starting treatment and is not related to the dosage of drug used. Sadly, although some improvement can be made after stopping the drug, most of the hair growth is irreversible and a permanent method of removal (electrolysis) is needed to remove these hairs.

b. Diazoxide

This drug is used in the treatment of high blood-pressure in adults and low blood sugar in children. In adults hair growth is rare (1 per cent) but in children it is common and occurs within six weeks of starting treatment. The areas affected are the face, back and extremities. The hair growth is completely reversible with cessation of the drug.

c. Minoxidil

This new drug is used in the treatment of high blood-pressure, and causes increased body hair in all patients within weeks of starting the drug. The hair is most prominent on the arms and face, and can be quite marked. Its effects are, however, reversible.

THE EXAMINATION

The extent of the examination depends upon what the doctor discovered from the questions asked.

The examination will involve 'grading' your body hair, i.e. determining which areas of your body are affected and by how much. This is important for three reasons:

1. Hair in certain areas (back, shoulders, neck, cheek, chest and abdomen – not in the mid-line) almost inevitably means there is a hormonal imbalance.
2. By knowing how hairy a woman is before a particular treatment is commenced, the doctor can assess the efficacy of the treatment.
3. Before any treatment is undertaken, the extent of body hair can be monitored over a period of time (usually six months) to see if the hair growth is worsening, as the woman believes it is.

An assessment will be made of weight and blood-pressure, and the presence and extent of acne will be noted. Signs of virilization will be sought (increased muscle mass, deepened voice, loss of breast tissue, balding over the temples, and lastly an increase in the size of the clitoris), as well as signs of excess cortisol or growth hormone (fat distribution increased especially over the face and upper back; large features, feet and hands, purple stretch marks over the body).

The doctor will also make an assessment of the size of your uterus and ovaries. He or she will do this by performing a *bimanual examination* (one hand on your lower abdomen pressing down against the other hand, which is inserted into and pushing up from your vagina). This is important in establishing whether or not your reproductive system feels normal.

THE INVESTIGATIONS

The number and kinds of tests the doctor performs depends on what was found from the questions and examination. Sophisticated tests will be performed by hospital doctors, but GPs also commonly carry out some tests on women with excess body hair. These include:

- Serum testosterone
  This is the most frequently performed test. The normal
  level of serum testosterone is between 0.2 and 0.8 mg/ml.
  It has been found that overall, up to 60 per cent of
  women who have excess body hair have normal
  testosterone levels. Of the women who have excess body
  hair and normal menstrual cycles, about 80 per cent have
  normal testosterone levels. In the women with normal
  testosterone levels, the cause of increased body hair will
  be one of the factors discussed on page 33.
  Of the remaining women with increased testosterone, the
  majority will still be normal, but will produce slightly
  higher than average levels, as also described on page 33.
  Only a very small minority of these women will have
  grossly elevated levels which would suggest an underlying
  illness.
- Serum DHEA-S, ACTH and Prolactin
  These tests will reveal an abnormality in the secretion of
  hormones from the adrenal or pituitary glands; they are
  only infrequently performed by GPs.
- Pelvic scan
  An ultrasound or similar scan of the pelvis will reveal the
  size of the ovaries, and thus will be able to eliminate the
  possibility that any increase in size is due to cysts or
  growths.

Medical Treatment for Women with Excess Body Hair and No Underlying Disease

The vast majority of women with excess body hair will have
no underlying abnormality even if a small number may have
raised testosterone levels. Some of these women have so much
body hair (or perceive that they have so much hair) that their

psychological well-being is damaged and their daily lives greatly affected. Other women can have the same amount of body hair, but as they do not perceive this as a problem can live a psychologically healthy and full life. Those women who are unable to cope with their body hair can turn to medical treatment, as well as cosmetic treatment, to reduce it.

There are two ways that these hair-reducing drugs work:

1. By decreasing the production of testosterone in the body, or
2. by preventing the testosterone from having its usual effect on the hair follicle cells.

With this reduction in testosterone (or the effectiveness of testosterone) the hair follicles slowly, step by step with each new growth cycle, become reduced in size, and the hair they produce becomes finer, slower growing and shorter. However, the hairs will never disappear completely, because once a hair and its follicle have converted to the larger terminal type, they cannot revert back to the vellus type.

There are a few basic characteristics that apply to all these hair-reducing drugs:

- They take about three months before they start having an effect.
- They take between nine and twelve months to achieve their full effect, after which there is little further improvement.
- The most noticeable improvement is on the trunk and limbs, especially the legs.
- Thick facial hair usually does not respond well to treatment.
- Any associated acne will usually improve.
- Other methods of hair removal are usually still necessary, although the frequency of their use is reduced.

- They have to be taken constantly for the hairs not to grow. As soon as treatment is stopped the level or effect of testosterone returns, and in the majority of women the hairs begin to grow again. It takes about six to nine months for the hair to return to pre-treatment levels.

There follows a description of these drugs:

Oral Contraceptives

The combined oral contraceptive pills contain two hormones; an oestrogen and a progestogen. There are many different kinds of combined oral contraceptives on the market, and they differ in both the kinds of oestrogen and progestogen used and the quantities of each.

Those that have been shown to reduce body hair contain the following hormones:

- Oestrogens
  ethinyloestradiol (30 to 50 µg) or mestranol (50 µg).
- Progestogens
  norethinderone (= norethisterone; 0.5 to 1 mg) or ethynodiol diacetate (1 mg).

The progestogens to be avoided because of their androgenic effects are: norgestrel, norethisterone acetate, and levonorgestren.

If you are already taking an oral contraceptive, the type of oestrogen and progestogen which it contains can usually be found on the side of the packet. Your doctor should be willing to change your prescription if it is unsuitable.

The effective oral contraceptives have reduced hair growth in 50 to 75 per cent of women, such that they can reduce their usage of temporary methods of hair removal. In 30 per cent of these women there is sufficient reduction in hair growth that other means of hair removal are unnecessary.

The possible side-effects are the same for any combined

oral contraceptive: lassitude, reduced libido, malaise, depression, weight gain, raised blood-pressure, and increased risk of thrombosis.

Oral contraceptives should not be used by women with a history of thrombosis or embolic disease, with hypertension, who smoke, or who are over 35.

Spironolactone

This drug acts by decreasing the level of testosterone and by preventing its entrance into hair follicle cells. About 70 per cent of women experience decreasing amounts of body hair.

It should not be taken by women who are pregnant, and must be prescribed only if the woman is taking adequate contraceptive protection. Often it is given successfully in combination with one of the oral contraceptive pills that also reduce hair.

The most common side-effect is heavy menstrual bleeding. This can be reduced by prescribing it cyclically (from day 4 to 21 of the menstrual cycle) or by prescribing it with an oral contraceptive. Women also complain of increased urine production, but this returns to normal after a few months.

Cyproterone Acetate

This drug (known as *Dianette* in the pharmaceuticals market) is widely used in Europe; it has not yet however been approved for use in the USA.

It has a number of actions which reduce the level and effectiveness of testosterone[3].

---

[3] It reduces the amount of testosterone made by the ovaries, increases the proportion of inactive, bound testosterone in the blood and also reduces the conversion, in the hair follicle cells, of testosterone to the specific hair-promoting androgen, *dihydrotestosterone*

It is made by only one drug company, and is prepared for use as an oral contraceptive[4].

It was originally prepared for the treatment of acne; when it was found to have the effect of reducing body hair it was also prescribed for that purpose.

It has been 70 per cent successful in reducing body hair, and a small number of women stopping the drug have not experienced a return to their pre-treatment levels of body hair.

The side-effects and contraindications are the same as for the oral contraceptives.

Underlying Diseases that Cause Excess Body Hair

I have already mentioned that only 1 per cent of the women with excess body hair who approach their doctors have any underlying disease. These diseases all cause a hormonal imbalance in the body; it is this imbalance, for one reason or another, that leads to hair growth. All these underlying diseases can be detected and treated; hair growth will diminish with treatment but will usually not disappear completely.

POLYCYSTIC OVARIAN DISEASE (OR SYNDROME)

This is the most common cause of hirsutism in women with an underlying hormonal imbalance. Women usually complain of excess body hair and reduced frequency of their menstrual cycle (i.e. bleeding much less often than monthly). Other possible symptoms include: no menstrual cycle at all, infertility, obesity, and acne. The disease is quite variable in the way it begins, and it is possible to have almost any combination

---

[4] By the addition of an oestrogen.

of the above symptoms. On examination the doctor may find that the woman's ovaries are enlarged – this would be the result of the presence of multiple cysts within them. These cysts are simply fluid-filled sacs, and are nothing to do with cancer. How this disease occurs and why is unknown, but other than the symptoms it presents with, it leads to no other problems.

The treatment depends on the symptoms. If reduction in body hair (and acne) is desired, then any of the drugs that were described for use by women with no underlying disease can be used with similar success rates (i.e. certain oral contraceptives, *spironolactone* and *cyproterone acetate*). If pregnancy is desired, *clomiphene citrate* is prescribed, but this will not treat the symptom of increased body hair.

OTHER DISEASES

The other diseases that can cause an increase in body hair are all extremely rare, and are listed below. If you would like to find out more about them, I suggest you either ask your GP or visit your local library.

- Cushing's disease
- testosterone-releasing cancers
- congenital adrenal hyperplasia
- acromegally
- thyroid disease (in children)

3

TEMPORARY METHODS OF
HAIR REMOVAL

Introduction

This chapter will deal with the different non-permanent methods of hair removal which are available to us, and will include: ingredients of these products where relevant, the way they work (including a discussion of their advantages and disadvantages), any side-effects and/or long-term problems they can produce, and where possible ways of minimizing these side-effects and problems.

There have been very few studies carried out that have either asked women questions about what they think of the different ways of hair removal or looked objectively at advantages, disadvantages and long-term effects of these methods. In November 1966, the British consumer report *Which?* ran a study on the effectiveness of different home depilatory products (creams, abrasives and waxes) and of electrolysis, by asking a large sample of women to try them out and express their opinions. In 1981 an electrolysis clinic in Toronto, Canada opened to the public and offered its services to women with excess facial and neck hair. The clinic is run by a dermatologist and his team, and since its opening they have collected and published data from their own observations and from responses to questionnaires on the subject of hair removal from the face and neck. In 1990 I carried out a questionnaire asking women about their experiences of hair removal. The questionnaires were given to women at a local beauty salon in the south of England.

Other than this handful of useful reports, I have not found any others which could benefit women in their pursuit of improving the methods of removing excess body hair. If you do not live in Britain it may be worth looking at consumer reports from your own country to see if tests have been run on the different epilation and depilation methods and brands available to you.

You have probably already tried out a number of methods of hair removal, and I've no doubt that you have abandoned some of them because of their distressing side-effects or lack of effectiveness. But how much time have you taken over trying to understand why a particular method was ineffective, or why you developed a problem with it, or how to minimize this problem? This chapter should give you some insight into these questions, and I hope that you will learn to improve the effectiveness of hair removal methods by your own experimentation as well as by my advice.

There are two ways of disguising body hair:

1. Bleaching it
2. Covering it up with make-up

There are three ways of removing body hair:

1. Depilation, where the hair shaft is removed and the hair follicle remains intact.
2. Epilation, where the hair shaft and the follicle are removed together.
3. Electrolysis, where the hair follicle is destroyed permanently, thereby preventing hair growth.

Disguise

BLEACHING

This is an excellent way of making dark hairs less visible. It can be used on all types of body hair, but most frequently is used on facial hair, especially above the upper lip (remember in the film *A Fish Called Wanda* when Jamie Lee Curtis is rushing around in her bedroom with cream bleach above her upper lip?).

Ingredients

The active ingredient that bleaches the hair is *hydrogen peroxide*. This solution can be bought in chemists in its pure form at different strengths, but usually either 3 per cent or 6 per cent (which is also called '20' or '10' by volume) is used for body hair bleaching. Strengths above 6 per cent are not recommended for this use. By itself it acts slowly, so commercially it is packaged with a small amount of ammonia (or another alkaline substance) to speed up the dissolving process; also added is a 'bleaching booster' such as *sodium peroxide* (or another persulphate) to speed up the bleaching process. Fragrances are also sometimes added to these ingredients. Commercial hair bleach is bought either as a solution or powder of hydrogen peroxide which you add to a cream or paste. Sometimes included are a spatula, mixing plate, or brush.

How Bleaches Work

The hair itself is mainly made up of dead keratinized cells; mixed within these cells is the hair pigment, called melanin. The best way to think of this pigment is as little packets of colour scattered throughout the hair shaft. The melanin pigment is of two types: *eumelanin*, which produces brownish and black hair colours, and *pheomelanin*, which produces reddish and orangey hair colours. A hair can differ both in the amount of each type of melanin it contains and the proportions of each, so that all hair colours from light blond to black are made by containing different amounts of each. For example, blond hair may have only a little bit of eumelanin and a negligible amount of pheomelanin, brown hair will have more eumelanin, with perhaps more pheomelanin if it has red highlights, black hair will have lots of eumelanin and perhaps lots of pheomelanin (or very little), red hair has got lots of pheomelanin and little eumelanin.

When eumelanin (the black/brown pigment) has hydrogen peroxide added to it, it bleaches easily to a pale yellow. However, pheomelanin (the red/orange pigment) hardly bleaches at all in the presence of hydrogen peroxide or the other bleaching agents added to commercial preparations. So, if you have red hair, bleaching will hardly have any effect on its colour. But, maybe more importantly, if you have brown hair with red highlights, bleaching it will remove only the brown colour and thus leave your hair much redder.

There is a predictable sequence of colour change when you add hydrogen peroxide to hair, and this sequence represents the gradual bleaching out of the eumelanin pigment. For example, a black hair containing only eumelanin will change first from black to brown, then to red, then orange, then gold, then yellow, and finally to pale yellow. This process can be interrupted at any point simply by removing the bleach before the full colour change has occurred.

Bleach also softens hair (I do not know how), which may explain why after bleaching a large area, for example your arm or thigh, the hairs feel finer.

Obviously, because hair continues to grow, within a few days you will notice the dark roots coming through.

Application

Usually the bleach solution or powder is mixed with the paste or cream and is spread thickly onto the area to be bleached. Every hair and all its shaft has to be covered in order for it all to be bleached. This mixture is left on for an allotted amount of time and is then wiped off. There is almost inevitably some reddening of the skin after this procedure, but it does not last very long. The process can be repeated often for body hair (but for head hair bleaching too frequently leads to its becoming damaged and lifeless).

Problems and Side-effects

Ineffectiveness
One common complaint is that the bleach hasn't changed the colour of the hair enough or at all. There are several reasons for this.

1. You are not leaving the bleach on for long enough. Although the instructions will give you a time limit after which you should remove the bleach, if you are not suffering any irritation it is acceptable to leave it on for a little longer. Your hair may have more pigment than average and thus need more bleaching time.
2. The bleach is not strong enough. For the same reason as above you may need a stronger bleach. You can add a little more of the bleach powder or solution to the paste, or you can use a stronger bleach solution (but not more than 6 per cent). Again, it is irritation of the skin that should limit the strength you use.
3. You have a lot of the red pheomelanin pigment in your hair. As I have mentioned, this pigment is fairly unbleachable, and so there is no effective way of bleaching this hair.

Hair Bleached Too Light
This can happen if you leave the bleach on for too long for your hair type. For example, if you have not got much pig-

ment in your hair it will not need the full bleaching time suggested. You will have to adapt your timing; put it on, then after a few minutes scrape off a little and see what colour your hair is. If it is pretty much invisible, it suggests that the colour matches your skin colour, so you can take it all off. If it still looks too dark, reapply bleach to that area and have another look a little later, etc. Hair (especially the moustache) looks less visible if it is a bit darker than the skin rather than a bit lighter.

Irritation

There are two possible causes for this.

1. Your skin may be sensitive to caustic (alkaline) substances, and the place where you applied the bleach may, as a result, become red and sore. You can check for this beforehand by applying a small amount to a test area first (the back of your wrist, for example) and waiting for a reaction. If there is one, you can try reducing the strength of the bleach. Otherwise you could try a different product, because they differ in alkalinity and the products they contain.
2. Sometimes when using powder bleach, the small granules of hydrogen peroxide do not fully dissolve in the cream, so that when applied to the skin they cause a little caustic burn which leaves a temporary white mark. You can prevent this by making sure the granules are adequately mixed together and dissolved.

Allergic Reaction
Very occasionally people have been allergic to the persulphate ('the booster') or to the fragrances added. The allergic reaction can be mild, e.g. generalized or localized itching with a rash, or, rarely, more severe, with chest tightening (asthma attack), fainting or shock. The more severe reactions are very rare.

If you have suffered any type of allergic reaction with their use, I suggest you do not use bleach again, or consult your GP before another attempt.

Advantages

- A 'natural' way of dealing with hair you don't want seen
- Avoids the many problems with regrowth
- Depending upon how much dark root you don't mind being visible, the bleaching can last from days to weeks

Disadvantages

- Some women find that, as the hair continues to grow, the mixture of dark roots and light tips looks very untidy
- Takes time to do and is a messy and slightly smelly procedure
- It is not cheap if large areas are to be done frequently

MAKE-UP

This is very useful, and can be very effective for disguising, for example, beard stubble. It can be bought at a cosmetic or pharmacist counter, but may also be supplied under the NHS as a cover-up solution if you have a severe problem. If you buy it from a cosmetic or pharmacy counter it may be worth revealing your intended use to the beautician or pharmacist, because he or she will often know the limitations of the products and how best to use them. One medical powder called *Eckosan* has proved quite effective.

Depilation

This is removal of the hair shaft without removing the hair follicle.

SHAVING

I must first and foremost say and stress what is uppermost in my mind: shaving does not, I repeat does not increase your hair's thickness, its rate of growth or its darkness, neither on your body nor on your face. It in no way alters the characteristics of the growth of that hair. Several scientific studies, on both human hair and animal hair, have been carried out to verify whether the oft-quoted stories about shaving making your hair grow faster, darker or thicker are true or not. None have so far come up with any evidence that they are true. And indeed, when we consider all that is known about hair growth, there is no reason to suppose that shaving should alter anything, just as cutting your nails does not alter the characteristics of your nail or its growth.

There are several reasons why people believe shaving does change the hairs:

1. The natural, uncut hair over the body grows initially as a very fine tip and only gradually gets thicker as it grows in length. (This is why with waxing the new hair growth is always so soft, because these short new hairs are very fine; it is only as they get longer that they reach their normal thickness). If these fine-tipped hairs are shaved, they become blunt and thicker-tipped, and thus feel thicker and coarser, however they are no thicker than that of a normal hair shaft at its base. They do not become thicker than your normal hair (see Figure 6).
2. They are perceived as being darker because instead of a mixture of light tips (because they are thinner) and dark bases over the area of hair, you only have dark bases. So the area is darker, but not because the hairs themselves are becoming darker than their normal colour.
3. People forget or do not realize that our bodies get hairier as we get older (except after the menopause, see page

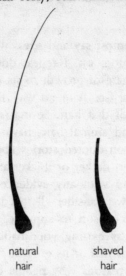

natural   shaved
hair   hair

Figure 6: Differences in the tips of natural and shaved hair

30). So if you have been shaving for years and complain
about increased hair growth and thickness, it has nothing
to do with shaving. You would have become hairier
naturally anyway.

I hope I have convinced you all that shaving does not affect
hair growth.

Uses

The Face and Neck
Women with thick hair in this area often have difficulties
bringing themselves to shave it. This seems to be for three
main reasons:

1. Women believe that by shaving their facial hair it will
   become stronger and thicker. This is not true, as I have
   explained above.

2. A lot of women feel that shaving the face is too masculine an act, and cannot bring themselves to do it. They would prefer to suffer the social consequences of thick facial hair than to shave. If a woman is not emotionally affected by her facial hair, or has very little hair there, then not shaving is understandable. But if the facial hair causes her terrible anguish and grief, I find it a tragedy that the act of shaving is such an insurmountable barrier. One of the surveys described how some women's lives were changed overnight once they started shaving.

3. Women are still being told by their GPs and their electrologists that they should not shave. If you are having electrolysis, it is actually beneficial to shave at the same time, as I shall explain later.

The Body

Shaving other parts of the body is an extremely common method of hair removal, and does not seem to produce many difficulties.

Shaving and Electrolysis

If you are having electrolysis on any part of the body or face, and the amount of hair in that area is not yet being kept to an acceptable level by the electrolysis, then it is absolutely fine, and even beneficial, to use shaving as a means of keeping hair growth under control. The only stipulation is that you leave between one and two days' growth on the area before you have each session of electrolysis (so that the hair and its direction of growth can be seen by the electrologist).

The reason it is beneficial to shave is because only hairs that are in their growth phase are successfully electrolysed (see page 105), so it is a waste of electrolysis time and money to remove hairs while they are in their resting phase. If you shave a few days before each electrolysis session, the electrologist will have a sample of growing hairs to choose from, as all the resting hairs will still be at skin level. Since about 70 per cent of hairs on the legs and 40 per cent of hairs on the face are resting, you would save yourself a lot of money and time, as well as having less visible hair, if you shave in concordance with electrolysis.

Electric Razors

Of all women that shave, about 30 per cent of them use this type of razor. The one disadvantage that all electric razors have in relation to safety ones is the reduced closeness of the shave.

Safety Razors

About 70 per cent of women prefer the safety razor, mainly because the shave is that much closer. You will achieve the best results if you soak the hair for a couple of minutes in warm water before shaving, to soften it. Also use lots of soap (with only a little water) or foam to make the shave smooth. Then, making sure you have good lighting, shave at your leisure.

In both methods of shaving one way of reducing facial stubble is to shave at least an hour or more after waking. This allows any fluid collection in the face (caused by sleeping horizontally) to drain down to your body, making your face less puffy and thus allowing a closer shave.

Problems and Side-effects

Cuts and Nicks

These can be avoided by using the precautions mentioned above. One person remarked that putting Chap Stick lip balm (it had to be this brand, she said) onto the cut seemed to promote healing – since hearing this I have learnt that cuts and grazes do actually heal several times faster if they have a layer of Vaseline (or equivalent) over the broken skin. Other women put a tiny piece of paper onto the cut, and some splashed a weak solution of *Eau de Cologne* over it. There is no doubt that some safety razors cut and nick skin far more than others, so it is worth trying out different brands if you find that you are suffering from this problem.

Irritation

Sensitive skin does suffer with shaving; this is caused by the uppermost layer of skin cells being scraped off as you shave. It can be minimized by making sure that the hairs have been softened and the shave is as smooth as possible (i.e. use lots of soap or foam), so that instead of the razor scraping cells off the skin it slides off them leaving them intact. A mild moisturizer used afterwards also helps. One woman found that using a loofah (or other mild abrasive) before shaving reduced the irritation by releasing the newly growing hairs from under the skin and making the skin smoother.

Razor Bumps (Pseudofolliculitis Barbae)

These are ingrowing hairs that sometimes occur over the face when the hair type is coarse and curly. What happens is that the hair grows out of the skin but then re-enters it again because of the sharp tip and its curly nature. The hair then continues to grow under the skin, compacting itself and developing into a small bump or spot which sometimes gets infected. It often happens in black skin where the hairs are especially curly. These bumps are then in danger of being nicked and made worse with continued shaving (see Figure 7).

One way of minimizing razor bumps is by using a depilatory cream instead of shaving. The rationale behind this is that depilatory creams leave the hair tips softer and not blunt-ended, thus the tips are less likely to re-enter the skin.

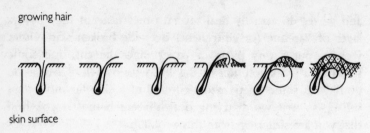

Figure 7: Development of a razor bump

However, the creams on sale in the European market are not strong enough to dissolve very coarse hair (see page 68).

Ingrowing Hairs
There are several types of ingrowing hairs; they will be discussed under the section on Waxing (see page 75).

Facial Stubble
I have already mentioned that facial stubble can be reduced if you shave more than an hour after waking so that your facial puffiness has gone, allowing the shave to be that much closer.

Advantages

- A fast, clean, easy and odourless way of removing body hair
- Cheap
- Particularly convenient if you are an allergic type of person
- Very useful in conjunction with electrolysis
- Does not distort the hair follicle in any way (see page 80).

Disadvantages

- Usually has to be done daily if the hair growth is thick, because the regrowth is so stubbly
- Other problems that can occur, as mentioned above.

TRIMMING

Some women have found that they prefer simply trimming certain areas of hair instead of shaving them and suffering the problems of ingrowing hairs. For example, bikini line hair, or hair at the back of thighs and pubic region. Obviously, trimmed hair does not feel as pleasant as that of a smooth shave, but then a spotty area does not feel particularly nice either.

DEPILATORY CREAMS

Uses

These creams (or foams or gels) are used for hair removal over almost any part of the body (however, thick beard growth is pretty resistant to them, see below).

Ingredients

The active ingredient is one of a number of the salts of *thioglycolic acid*, usually *calcium thioglycolate*. This salt needs a high alkaline environment to be effective, and so an alkaline chemical is added, usually *calcium* or *sodium hydroxide*. Because these ingredients tend to smell fairly bad, a fragrance is added to the product to make it more acceptable (some products seem to have achieved a much more acceptable smell than others). Sometimes a finishing cream, a soothing cream or a moisturizer is included. There is also occasionally a spatula or applicator provided.

Cosmetics and pharmaceuticals companies have made the creams for use in different areas, thus some creams are stronger than others.

In some countries (for example in Latin America) it is still possible to buy a depilatory cream which is much stronger than those available in Britain (and which does in fact easily remove coarse facial hair). The active ingredient of these creams is either strontium sulfide or barium sulfide. You can recognize these creams because their smell is absolutely and utterly foul (hydrogen sulfide gas, for instance, which smells of rotten eggs), especially when in contact with water. However hard you try, you cannot get away without experiencing some unpleasant smells. It is this smell which limits their use and has led to their being withdrawn from the markets in Britain and North America.

How Depilatories Work

The thioglycates are in fact the same chemicals as those found in home-perm solutions, but for hair removal they are much stronger. In home-perm solutions the weak thioglycate acts by breaking only some of the chemical bonds within the hair shaft and then allowing the hair to become fixed in a different position, usually with a wave. With the depilatory creams the process goes one step further – so many bonds are broken within the hair that it becomes very weak and eventually disintegrates. These thioglycate depilatories have been produced as an aqueous solution, so that as the hair breaks down it absorbs water and becomes jelly-like and is therefore easy to wipe away. The depilatories also penetrate the hair follicle a little deeper than the skin surface, so that hair below this surface is also dissolved. Thus it takes about one to two days after removal before new hair growth is detectable above the skin. The disintegration of the hair does not leave the tip of the hair blunt (as in shaving) but rather fine, so new growth feels softer.

Because of the close similarity between what skin is made of and what the hair shaft is made of, any chemical that destroys hair will also be able to destroy skin. So it is very important to follow the package instructions carefully and not leave the cream on for longer than is recommended. This is also the reason why it is strongly suggested that you try out the cream on a small test area beforehand. If you do not suffer any irritation you can continue.

Application

The cream (or gel or foam) is applied in a thick layer onto your skin. It should not be allowed to dry out, because if it does so it will lose its effectiveness. Depending upon the make, it is left on for between five and twenty minutes, and should not be left on for any longer than is recommended.

In addition, these products should only be used on healthy skin; any spots, cuts, eczema or other skin conditions that lead to broken skin should not be in contact with the cream. (Think of your skin as a barrier against harmful chemicals. If it is broken in any way these chemicals can reach sensitive, susceptible tissue below and cause damage). If you have any doubts ask your GP.

Problems and Side-effects

Contact Allergy

The thioglycates and the fragrances added have been known to cause contact allergy in some people, i.e. some time after applying it to the skin the area becomes red and inflamed and may become itchy. If you have this problem you could try another cream, since you might be allergic to the fragrance and not the thioglycolate. You may find, however, that no cream suits you.

Irritant Dermatitis

Some people have skins that are very sensitive and that easily develop a rash when exposed to chemicals (such as those found in washing-up liquid or cream cleaners). Such women will not be able to leave the product on for long enough for it to be effective. In fact, if the product is left on for too long anyone would develop this kind of rash.

If a rash occurs it can be soothed with a cool wet wash-cloth and calamine lotion or a gentle moisturizer. Adding alcohol (for example *Eau de Cologne*) will only irritate it further.

Ingrowing Hairs
These are particularly common around the bikini and upper thigh areas, and are discussed under Waxing (see page 83).

Coarse Hair Not Removed
The thicker and coarser your hair is the more hair material there is to dissolve. Make sure you have put a thick layer of cream over such areas, and that the cream has not dried out. Keep it on for the longest recommended time. If it still does not dissolve it might be worth trying a different product, because as I have mentioned, different ones have got different strengths. The only other solution is to find the cream made of *strontium sulfide* or *barium sulfide*, which as I have explained is a much more effective (albeit smelly) product for thick hair.

Advantages

- Hair growth takes one or two days to reach the skin surface, and when it does it is much softer than the hair growth of shaved hairs
- There are of course no cuts or nicks

Disadvantages

- A messy way of removing hair, and despite fragrances never smells particularly nice
- The smell tends to linger for several hours
- More expensive than shaving and more time-consuming
- Skin irritation is not uncommon

ABRASIVES

These are usually used over body hairs that are not too coarse.

Ingredients

Abrasives are made of a variety of stone-like materials; fine sand paper, emery paper, abrasive stones (e.g. pumice stone). They are shaped into either a block that you hold or incorporated into mittens that you slip onto your hand.

How Abrasives Work

They work in that by rubbing an area of hair it will eventually break off or be rubbed away at the skin surface. The finish is smooth, but when the hair grows back it feels quite rough (but not as stubbly as after shaving).

Problems and Side-effects

The major problem is irritation to the skin, because the rubbing action removes its uppermost layer of cells. The area can be treated with a cool washcloth and soothing moisturizer.

Advantages

- Useful if you are in a rush but have no time for a shower or bath!
- Neither messy nor time-consuming (unless the hair is fairly thick)
- The gloves seem to be more effective and easier to use than the blocks

Disadvantages

- The gloves wear out quite quickly, so it is not as cheap a method of hair removal as shaving
- Only fairly fine hair is successfully removed, because if it

is too thick, too much skin is rubbed off before the hair is removed, causing marked irritation

Epilation

This is the removal of the hair shaft with the hair bulb (or root).

PLUCKING AND TWEEZING[1]

Uses
This method is often used for removing small areas of hair (e.g. eyebrows, moustache, hair around the nipple area) or for the removal of the occasional lonely thick hairs found anywhere. Some women have used this method to clear very thick facial hair, but I hope to convince these individuals that plucking (or any other method of epilation) is strongly not recommended for removing thick facial hair.

Methods
Although one pair of tweezers is very much like any other, the way that people pluck differs greatly. Some pluck careful-ly, taking one hair out at a time and being careful to avoid pinching the skin. Then there are those that cannot resist pinching, squeezing, poking and persisting, even though the hair is determined not to be pulled out yet! And these people know full well that if they let the hair grow just a little longer the whole process would be hassle-free! Need it be mentioned which method is more likely to produce infec-tions, scabbing, ingrowing hairs and scarring?

It is true, however, that even the most carefully plucked

[1] Papers written on the effectiveness of plucking have mainly looked at the effects of removing thick hair on the face, neck and nipples.

area will have some post-plucking inflammation which looks red and lasts for hours.

Is good plucking any different from waxing? You are effectively doing the same thing, i.e. tearing out a hair from its follicle and causing a lot of surrounding tissue damage (for example, broken cells, torn nerve endings and ruptured blood vessels). Having looked at the research and literature on both methods I found that plucking often causes long-term ill effects (for example pitting and scarring) that waxing seems on the whole to have avoided. I believe that it is *not the method of hair removal* that leads to this difference, but rather *the different types of body hair*, which react differently. We are more likely to pluck some areas and wax others (see below).

Problems and Side-effects

Hyperpigmentation, Pitting and Scarring

If we look at the effects of plucking around the beard, moustache and neck area as compared to the nipple area we find a big difference. Around the nipple women very rarely get any post-plucking problems, and judging from the responses to my questionnaire women seem to have no problems with plucking along the abdominal and chest mid-line. However, it is a different story for beard, moustache and neck hairs: women with *coarse* facial hair are much more likely to develop pitting and scarring, whereas those with finer facial hair are able to repeatedly pluck (or wax) these hairs with no long-term effects. There is however some individual variation in the response to plucking different thicknesses of hair from the face. Furthermore, there can be a difference in the kind of hair regrowth in this area after plucking: some follicles develop long fine hairs, whereas others develop coarser hairs.

Why is there a difference in response to plucking in these facial areas as compared to other areas? I believe it is all related to the size of the follicle. In the male, beard, moustache and neck hairs are the *coarsest* on the whole body, and women, as we know, are able to grow hairs in this area as thick as those seen in men. The hair follicles of these coarse hairs are the largest in the body. This means that they have more blood vessels going to them, they have a larger nerve supply, and generally have more tissue around and attached to them.

I have already mentioned that removing a hair from its natural environment is equivalent to tearing the follicular and surrounding tissue, causing damage and inflammation. You can imagine that the larger the follicle the more damage will be caused; and the more damage there is, the longer it will take to heal, the more likely there is to be scarring, and the more likely it is that that follicle and the surrounding tissue will become distorted and abnormal after the initial healing has taken place. This is analogous to the healing process after a large deep cut compared to a smaller superficial one; small ones usually heal with no scarring, but big ones can leave you with a dent, a bump, extra pigmentation or slightly different skin. This is the why I believe that epilation of any relatively fine hair usually causes no long-term damage, whereas epilation of the coarse facial hair does.

I hope I have convinced all those who pluck (or epilate in any way) these coarse facial hairs that it is extremely unwise to do so. You would be much better off if you shaved this area if you want to clear it of hairs – or try shaving and electrolysis together (the benefits are described on pages 61 and 105–9). If, on the other hand, you have been plucking coarse facial hairs for years and you have not developed any scarring or pitting, etc., then you are one of the lucky few who heals well, and there is no reason why you cannot continue the way you are.

Ingrowing Hairs

These occur especially around the bikini line, and are discussed under Problems and Side-effects of Waxing (see page 83).

Distorted Roots

These are described under Problems and Side-effects of Waxing (see page 80).

Keloid Scars

Some skin types, notably black, develop keloid scars easily. If you have developed such scars (which look like little hard bumps of extra skin tissue) you are advised not to pluck or tweeze.

ELECTRIC EPILATING DEVICES

How They Work

Recently several companies have designed electric hand-held devices that pull out individual hairs when run up and down the area of skin (see Figure 8). The mechanism of action is usually two intertwined metal coils that rotate against one another, trapping hairs that come their way and then holding onto them until they are pulled out by their roots. The effect is like a very fast plucking machine, with one or two hairs being plucked out at any one time until the whole area is free of hair.

Problems and Side-effects

Problems such as inflammation and folliculitis, pain, and ingrowing hairs are all discussed in the section on Waxing (see next section).

Advantages

- A clean, very effective way of epilating hairs in your own home

- The machines are not too expensive, and once you have bought one there is no further cost (except for electricity)
- Not messy or smelly
- Can be done for a little bit of time on a few hairs (rather than the time-consuming total removal of hairs as with waxing)

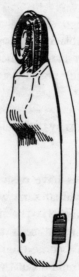

Figure 8: An electric hand-held epilation machine

Disadvantages

- Despite the claims of the advertisers, this is an incredibly painful procedure for a lot of women, and they sometimes have to stop using it for this reason. However, there is no doubt that you get accustomed to the pain with repeated use
- The hairs have to be at least ½ cm (¼ in) long for the machine to remove them, and it seems that the longer the hair is (above this length), the more painful it is to use the machine (or is it simply because if they are longer it

means you have not used the machine frequently enough and have not therefore become used to the pain, or have forgotten how bad it is?)
- Seems to be preferred in women who do not have very coarse hair (mainly I think because it is less painful). However, fine hair tends to break off in the metal coils rather than being pulled out properly.
- Can only be used easily on fairly large flat areas (like the legs)
- Is noisy and very time-consuming if you have lots of hairs

THREADING
This is an ancient technique still used extensively in some Saudi Arabian countries, and occasionally in Europe.

Method
The device used is simply a long piece of string. The woman twists it onto itself, then puts one end in her mouth and runs the other along her skin. The twisted string acts very much like the rotating coils in home epilating machines, in that it traps hairs between its threads and holds onto them until they have been pulled out. A lot of the hairs are also snapped off at the surface of the skin. The process is apparently painful, and must be as time-consuming as electric devices. The problems and side-effects are also no different from those with the electric device.

WAXING

Uses
Waxing is like mass plucking. It is used for removing large areas of hair (e.g. on the legs and arms) or distinct smaller areas (e.g. bikini line, fine facial hair). It is used in women who do not mind having regrowing hairs over their skin and

thus do not have a completely 'silky smooth' finish for a few weeks.

Ingredients

Waxes usually contain a mixture of resins, beeswax, oils and glucose. They also sometimes have perfumes added. The majority of waxes are solid at room temperature and are called 'hot' or 'warm' waxes. These have a low melting point, which means that they change to their liquid form at a warmish temperature (between the temperature of a warm or hot shower).

Another type of wax, used less often, is the cold wax, which is in liquid form at room temperature and does not harden. This type of wax usually comes out of a tube in a sticky liquid form.

The packaging can also contains strips of cloth, brush, spatula, pan, and/or post-wax soothing cream.

Another type is cold wax that already has its backing tape attached. You buy many sticky bits of tape ready for use (like very sticky plaster).

Application

Waxing can be done at home or in a beauty salon.

The solid wax is melted down in a metal pot (either provided or your own). Nowadays one can buy proper electrical wax melting pots that are used in salons; these are very useful if you have large areas to wax regularly, because they maintain an even temperature which is easily controlled — they are not cheap, however. The temperature should be kept only as high as necessary to melt the wax, so that it does not burn you when it is applied.

The area to be waxed is usually prepared by cleaning it with alcohol to remove any oils (natural or cosmetic moisturizers) that might prevent the wax sticking to the hairs; the skin is then sprinkled with talcum powder so that it is protected from sticking to the wax. The hairs must be at least ¼ cm (⅛ in) long so that the wax can stick well to them and pull them out.

Once the wax has melted (and the temperature should be checked over a small area beforehand to make sure it is not too hot), a layer is spread onto a small area of skin (by brush or spatula) and allowed to become more solid. When the wax is a thicker consistency (i.e. not tacky) it is pulled off quickly *against* the direction of the hairs. To do this a little corner is peeled away from the skin in order to get a good grip of the wax before pulling (a bit like pulling a plaster off your body).

With some waxes, instead of pulling the wax itself, a strip of cloth is pressed into the wax so that it sticks well to it and then both the cloth and wax are pulled off.

With cold waxes, since they do not solidify, they too have some kind of cloth put over them, which is then pulled off.

The type of wax that is already laid out on backing tape like a plaster you stick onto the area and pull off.

All the hairs that are embedded in the wax get pulled out from their roots. Very often when large areas of hair are waxed you can see tiny white casts coming out of each opening in the skin. These are the inner root sheaths of the hair follicle (see page 18), and means that the hairs have been pulled out when they are still growing. Other hairs will not be stuck well in the wax and thus do not get pulled out, still others are broken at the skin surface, and some are so strongly attached to their follicle (and these are inevitably hairs in their resting phase) that they do not get pulled out at all.

This action of spreading wax over a small area, letting it dry and then pulling it off is repeated over the whole area to be waxed. As your technique improves you can put wax over several areas and pull each bit off in sequence.

The more thorough beauticians will go over the waxed area with a pair of tweezers to remove any remaining hairs.

It does not sound difficult, but I have witnessed scenes at the end of waxing sessions where there has been wax all over the hands of the beautician as well as bits over the newly-waxed skin, the couch, and over the floor and on clothing! Cold waxes are particularly sticky and messy. There are other more difficult problems that can occur with home-waxing, so it might be a good idea for you to see how it is done properly in a salon before you attempt it alone.

The common salon waxing method is the one using no cloth, so that the wax can be remelted and reused many times. This means that the salon waxes used on your skin have been used before on other people, and their hair and bits of skin cells are all mixed up in the wax. This might turn some people's stomachs!

After the hairs have been pulled out, the remaining pores (where the hairs were) are open and initially vulnerable to infection. However, they naturally very quickly become small openings again, which are closed to the entry of bacteria. Some salons put weak alcohol solution onto the area, others a mild non-perfumed moisturizer.

Because the hairs have been pulled out by the roots it takes about 10 to 14 days for new hairs to reach beyond the skin surface. If you feel hairs on your skin before this time, these are the hairs that were either left in, were broken at the shaft or were at the skin surface at the time of waxing.

The new hair growth starts from the hair bulb, and the tips of these hairs are fine and gradually get thicker as they get longer. So this regrowth initially feels finer than your normal hair.

The amount and length of hair you allow to regrow depends upon how you feel about this hair being there at all. The only rule is that the hair must be at least ¼ cm (⅛ in)

long before the next waxing session. Some women do not
mind their hair being this length before they have it waxed
again; others want it removed as quickly as possible. The
average hair will grow about 1 cm (½ in) each month once
it is at the skin surface. So if you leave your hair for six
weeks after waxing it will be about 1 cm (½ in) long
(because it takes about two weeks to first reach the skin surface).

Problems and Side-effects

Inflammation and Folliculitis

As for plucking, no one gets away without some redness, and
a general rule is: the thicker the hair the more inflammation
there will be. Areas of fine hairs will usually become only
red, coarser hairs will leave a 'plucked chicken' effect (this is
folliculitis, which basically means inflammation of the follicle),
and really coarse hairs (for example those as thick as pubic
ones) might also leave a tiny speck of blood. These effects are
all caused because you have torn living tissue (the hair bulb
and the hair sheath) away from its living environment (the
hair follicle).

For some women, these effects can last up to two days, for
others only a few hours. The kind of reaction you get
depends on your skin type, as well as the coarseness of the
hair that has been removed.

There are two effective ways of reducing this problem;

1. An aspirin (or an equivalent drug; ask your GP about it)
    acts as an 'anti-inflammatory', and can be taken about one
    hour before the wax session and then repeated six to eight
    hours afterwards.
2. Hydrocortisone cream, at strengths of 0.5 per cent and 1
    per cent, are now available to the general public without a

prescription. This product, which is a steroid, is another
type of anti-inflammatory drug and is very effective.
Hydrocortisone, like aspirin, prevents or reduces
inflammation by, in medical terms, stopping part of the
body's natural response to injury around the injured site.
The injury will still heal, but with less inflammation. It is
applied sparingly to the area after waxing and worked in
until it has completely disappeared. Although it is a steroid
(and this might frighten some people), it is very weak, and
used sparingly will not cause any side-effects. The label on
the tube mentions that it should not be used excessively.

Both these methods usually reduce the inflammation enough
for the area to look presentable within a few hours.

Distorted Roots

Although no scientific studies have been done on the effects
of epilation on the root of the hair, it seems common knowledge that roots do become distorted the more you wax them
(see Figure 9). This means that hairs may begin to grow in
the wrong direction, leading to untidy growth or ingrowing
hairs; more importantly it makes the process of electrolysis
much more difficult, if you decide to have this done at a
later date (see page 109).

Infected Spots

Some people, especially with home-waxing, have experienced
infected, pus-filled spots in many of the follicles as soon as a
few hours after waxing. This is either because your technique
is unhygienic (for example using a dirty cloth after waxing to
dissolve or wash away remaining wax) or because you are
prone to infections. Either way they can be reduced by more
hygienic preparations; however, if you are prone to skin
infections even very sterile conditions may not be enough to
prevent these spots.

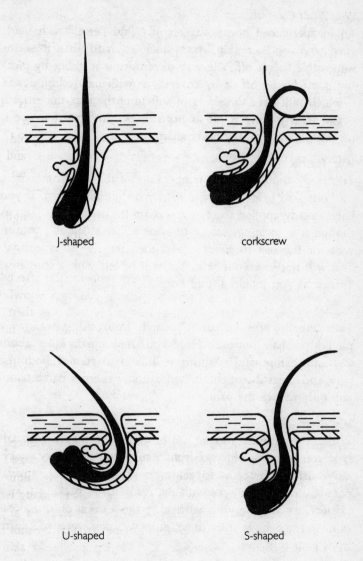

J-shaped

corkscrew

U-shaped

S-shaped

Figure 9: Four kinds of distorted hair follicles

Wax Won't Come Off

An inexperienced home-waxer could find herself with hard-ened wax on her skin, wax stuck so hard that it seems impossible to get off. The way to remove it is either by pick-ing it off bit by bit or by covering it with newly liquid wax – which will have the effect of softening the wax underneath – and then pulling it off as normal. Do not try to scrape it off with a knife or any other sharp utensil.

Wax Too Hot

You really should test the temperature of the wax somewhere on your skin before you spread any on the hairy area. If you have already applied too hot a wax on the area and it feels as though it is burning, scrape or wipe off as much as you can, wait for the rest to solidify, and then pull it off as normal. You will not lose your skin, but will be left with a sore area. Treat it as you would a mild burn.

Pain

This actually prevents some people from using wax as a method of hair removal. Have you tried a pain-killer about an hour beforehand? Aspirin will help to reduce both the pain and the subsequent inflammation, whereas paracetamol will only reduce the pain.

Mess

Without experience waxing can be incredibly messy, especial-ly if you use the cold wax from a tube, which is very sticky, never dries and seems to get everywhere. There are several possibilities: try the wax with the ready-made backing (like a plaster), try waxing with a friend, go to a salon on one occa-sion and see how it is done properly, persevere and learn from your mistakes.

Hyperpigmentation

Some women with darker skin suffer from hyperpigmentation in areas where ingrowing hairs have occurred. This is the darkening or increased pigmentation of an area of skin. The exact reason for it is unknown, but the resolution of the ingrowing hair usually reduces the pigmentation, albeit over a long period of time.

Ingrowing Hairs

The topic of ingrowing hairs deserves a whole chapter to itself. The number of women that experience this problem is enormous, and the amount of time, energy and distress that is caused is equally great.

There were many different descriptions of ingrowing hairs in the responses to my questionnaire, but I have tried to divide them into four main types (see Figure 10), relating to how they look and their management:

1. Those hairs that track along just under the skin surface, so that a thin dark line is visible under the skin.

   This type does not produce too much of a problem, because the area does not get infected, does not look bad and feels smooth. If these occur, you can either wait for them to reach the outside world (as most of them eventually do), or you can carefully nick the skin with a clean needle (a needle is sharper than a pin, and causes less trauma to the surrounding skin) and gently pull out the hair leaving it attached to its root. These ingrowing hairs can usually be prevented by moisturizing and using a loofah on the skin regularly (see below).

2. Those small hairs that are on areas of frequent pressure (for example the back of the thigh, the knees, elbows and the backside) that are too small to push themselves out of the follicle (which is clogged with compact debris (e.g. sebum) because of all the pressure applied there), and thus just curl around themselves under the skin in the follicle.

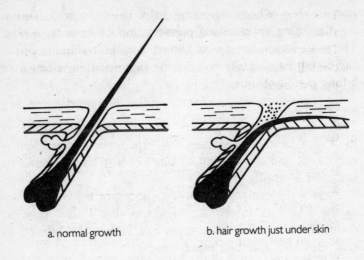

a. normal growth   b. hair growth just under skin

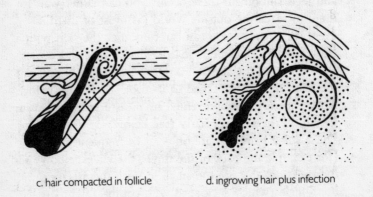

c. hair compacted in follicle   d. ingrowing hair plus infection

Figure 10: Types of ingrowing hairs

These hairs feel like goose pimples, usually start occurring about 10 to 14 days after waxing, and continue for weeks. They are neither infected nor filled with pus, and if you carefully dissect one you will find a tiny hair scrunched up and mixed in with a bit of dry material.

The way to minimize these, and it is quite effective, is to rub the area with a loofah or slightly rough sponge daily (either dry or while washing) and to follow this with moisturizer. This is best done twice a day, but once is also effective. This will remove some of the layers of dead skin cells, free such curled-up hairs, and soften the skin so that future hairs can reach the surface easily. You should start doing this right after having the waxing done, so as to prepare the skin for the hairs; continue it for several weeks, until all the hairs have reached the surface.

3. I have already described the ingrowing hairs one gets with shaving and known as 'razor bumps' (see page 63).
4. The biggest, most unsightly problem is the ingrowing hair associated with an infection.

These hairs, which are usually quite coarse, do not grow out of the skin but continue to grow underneath it and penetrate surrounding tissue (which does not normally have hairs within it – i.e. beyond the hair follicle). The body regards these hairs as foreign material, and an inflammatory reaction occurs around them (in the same way that a splinter causes inflammation if not removed) and attempts to digest and destroy them. At some stage during this development an infection may also establish itself, and the whole follicle becomes red, tender, angry and raised. Pus may eventually come to the surface, or the spot can continue without a visible head for weeks. There are several reasons for the occurrence of these ingrowing hairs:

- the hair follicle has been so deformed with repeated waxing that the natural direction of growth is not upwards and out but sideways, away from the hair follicle, so that the hair grows out of its natural environment
- the skin over the hair follicle is covered with a scab (or a plug of cells, oils and other material) so that the hair cannot push past it and instead grows around it and inwards
- these hairs are in areas of pressure and are thus prevented from growing out, for example they may be growing around the back of your thighs, or along the bikini line where either material, underwear elastic or thick skin prevents the normal direction of growth.

This last type of ingrowing hair is most severe in the bikini line and the pubic triangle. However, it is also seen over the front of thighs and the back of thighs or occasionally over the face if the hair is coarse. In the pubic region the hair is quite coarse (women with fine hairs in these areas usually do not complain about this problem), the skin is sometimes moist, well-covered and warm, and bacteria are plentiful and can easily penetrate pores and help establish an infection. Whether a pore gets slightly infected first and thus prevents the hair from growing out of the skin (and so establishes itself as an ingrowing hair) or whether an ingrowing hair leads to inflammation in the surrounding skin which is then more prone to infection, I do not know. It is probably a mixture of the two, but the effect is the same: an unsightly spot that can last for weeks. The size of the spot can vary from a fairly small one which is not much bigger than the follicle (and in these the ingrowing hair and pus is usually superficial enough to be visible), to spots that are so deep and large that areas as large as 3 cm (1½ in) in circumference become tender, raised and red, but without any pus or hair being visible.

These spots are so common there should be a warning about them when undergoing any kind of hair removal in this area!

There are several measures that can be taken to reduce these spots:

1. As already mentioned, a daily rub with a loofah (or its equivalent) followed by a moisturizer will prevent a lot of the little ingrowing hairs in this area by removing surface debris. Some women prefer to use a body scrub cream (made up of fine granules) – the net effect is the same.
2. It is important that this area is kept as clean, well-aired and as dry as possible.
3. Tight underwear elastic and tights would be better replaced with loose-fitting underwear and stockings.
4. The ingrowing hair and its associated infection will not resolve until either the hair has been digested or is removed. The body will eventually digest the hair, but it takes weeks to do so. As long as you can see the hair, or part of it, and you are fairly certain of not producing too much surrounding tissue damage, you can remove it by carefully picking it out with a clean needle and pulling it free. If it is attached to surrounding tissue I would leave it that way so that the follicle has time to heal with the hair in its natural place.

   If the hair is particularly long it means it has been growing under the skin for some time, and you will usually find it is thinner than a normal hair in this area and is often unattached to any surrounding tissue. This is because the process of digestion has already started. These hairs come out easily when pulled.

   Once the hair is out or in its natural place you will find that the whole spot will slowly heal. The area is however equivalent to that of a newly-squeezed spot, and will be susceptible to further infection. There are some local antibiotic creams that can be prescribed, but they should be used sparingly and selectively so that their effectiveness does not diminish through your skin building up resistance to them. The area should furthermore be kept dry and clean. One woman surveyed mentioned that regularly dabbing vitamin C powder over the spot really did seem to promote healing (although it stings very much when first applied, and turns the oozing fluid black). Vitamin C is used by the body for wound healing and is actually concentrated naturally in wounds.

5. When the spot is just a red, raised and very tender area but no hair can be seen, you are faced with a dilemma: either you poke around with a clean needle looking for the hair to set it free, or you leave it alone and let your body do the work by digesting it. Basically you will want to use the quickest method that allows healing to occur, but which method that is depends on the individual spot and the person. What is needed is a study where women leave one side of their bodies to nature and pick at the spots on the other side, and then see which is heals quicker. I shall have to leave you with the decision!

From the responses to the questionnaires it seems that some women are never free of these unsightly spots, and often have many of them.

There are several things that can be done if the above tips have not reduced the problem to an acceptable level:

1. It seems that the more of the hair shaft that is removed the more likely it is for the problem to develop. You should therefore think of changing your method of hair removal, just in the area where you have spots. Epilation causes more ingrowing hairs than depilation, and in

depilation, the creams produce more than shaving. Change to a method that is less likely to produce the problem. For example, change from waxing to depilatory creams, or from creams to shaving.

2. Some women have found that the only solution was to trim their hair, leaving just enough above the surface so that it did not look too visible, was not too bristly, and all the hairs were free from the possibility of growing underneath. It takes a good few months for a spot-ridden area to fully heal and all the hairs to be growing outwards as normal.

3. Bleach these hairs.

4. Think about having electrolysis in this area, which will eventually be permanent hair removal. While having it you will, of course, suffer ingrowing hairs, but they will reduce in number as the hairs thin out, and you can look forward to a hair-free area in future.

References

Boots & Co. Ltd, plc, *Depilatories*, 1990.

4

ELECTROLYSIS: A PERMANENT METHOD OF HAIR REMOVAL

Introduction

To date there is only one way of safely and permanently removing hair. This is by destroying the hair bulb using a method called *electrolysis*.

As described in Chapter 1, the hair bulb has in its base a core of germinating cells which have the potential and ability to grow a hair, just as a flowering bulb has the potential to grow a particular type of flower. Removing the hair by plucking or waxing will remove most of the hair bulb, but it will not remove these germinating cells, which can divide and differentiate into a hair and its associated tissues. As long as these cells are in place and working there remains the potential for hair growth, and even after many growth cycles these cells remain and continue to produce new hairs (just as a flowering bulb has the potential to develop one flower after another but still remains a bulb, i.e. a separate functioning unit). These germinating cells have to be removed or destroyed in order for a hair follicle to lose its ability to grow a hair. The only method so far developed that can destroy these cells is electrolysis.

The goal of electrolysis is to destroy the bulb of the hair without disrupting the surrounding skin. The result of electrolysis is a hair follicle that is no longer able to grow a hair, with the skin surrounding the follicle left undamaged.

The word electrolysis has been modified through the years to describe any method of hair root destruction that uses a needle to discharge a destructive electric current (see below). As I shall describe, there are several types of currents which can be used, and although each has a specific scientific name, the blanket term for all of them is electrolysis.

Methods

Electrolysis is performed as follows:

1. A fine needle is inserted into the hair follicle until it reaches the hair bulb. This is by necessity a 'blind' procedure, because it takes place below the surface of the skin (see Figure 11).
2. Some kind of destructive electric current is then passed through the needle (from an instrument called an *epilation machine*) and is discharged into the tissues of the hair root and bulb. While this current is being discharged the client will experience a strange sensation, ranging from definite pain to just a tingle, depending upon the individual.
3. The needle is then removed, and the hair, which should now be free of its attachments to surrounding tissue within the follicle, is pulled out easily with tweezers.

The current passed will damage hair follicle tissue, hair root and the bulb tissue. Some of the bulb tissue will contain the germinating cells. If enough damage has occurred to the germinating cells they will be destroyed, and the hair follicle will have no potential for new hair growth and will remain 'hairless' for the rest of its days. If not enough damage has occurred to the germinating cells they will still have the potential to grow a hair, and will do so, although it might be

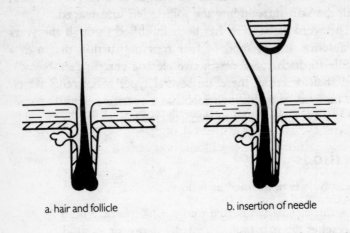

a. hair and follicle   b. insertion of needle

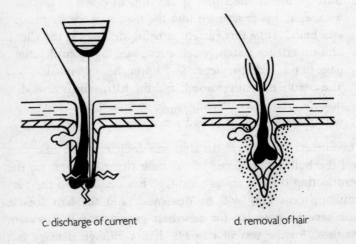

c. discharge of current   d. removal of hair

Figure 11: Electrolysis

finer or in some way different from the original one. This new hair growth is called *regrowth*, and is an important factor in assessing the effectiveness of electrolysis (see page 103). The client will continue to have electrolysis until gradually the hair becomes sparser and less electrolysis is needed. Eventually all the hair follicles in the treated area will have lost the ability to grow hair.

There are at present three methods of electrolysis which are recognized by the medical profession as ways of permanently removing hair: galvanic electrolysis, thermolysis, and 'the blend'.

GALVANIC ELECTROLYSIS

This was the first method of electrolysis developed, and was initially used by a physician in 1875 for the treatment of 'ingrowing eyelashes'. It uses direct electric current, discharged from the needle to the tissues and causing tissue damage by means of a 'chemical burn' (it is in fact a caustic burn)[1].

The current is discharged from all parts of the needle which are in contact with a moist environment (i.e. from the skin surface to the bulb – see Figure 12). This type of electrolysis needs at least a minute of discharging current before enough has been emitted for destruction to occur. This can be recognized by the appearance of tiny white bubbles of hydrogen gas around the base of the hair. The main drawback of this method is the time that the needle has to stay in position within the follicle while discharging its current,

[1] What actually happens is that the electrons from the needle tip enter the surrounding hair follicle tissue and convert the water and salt in this tissue to hydrogen gas and sodium hydroxide. The hydrogen gas escapes, and the sodium hydroxide, which is an alkaline substance, causes a caustic burn to the tissues it comes into contact with. $H_2O + NaCl \rightarrow H_2 + NaOH + Cl^-$

which, as mentioned, is at least a minute. Although of the three methods of electrolysis this is the surest one of producing permanent hair removal, it is not often used because of the time taken for each hair treatment.

There have been a couple of modifications to this method. One is the use of a multiple needle, where up to 16 needles

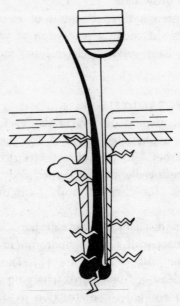

Figure 12: Discharge of current along the length of hair root and bulb

are used, placing and removing the needles in different follicles and always maintaining several discharging needles at any one time. This technique is not often used, however, because other methods (mentioned below) are so much easier for the operator. Another, more recent modification has been the design of an insulated needle, so that all the discharging current occurs at the very tip of the needle and thus damages only the very bottom of the hair bulb, where the

germinating cells are. There have, as yet, been very few studies to show whether this needle is more effective than the
standard needle which discharges current along its length, but
results have been positive so far.

THERMOLYSIS

Since its development in 1924 this mode of electrolysis has
taken over from the previous one because of its speed of
action. Other names for this type of electrolysis are: short-
wave electrolysis and, more frequently, diathermy.

Thermolysis uses indirect high-frequency electric current to
heat up the water particles in the moist follicular environment. Temperatures of up to 200°F (93°C) are generated,
and it is this high temperature which causes local tissue damage and leads to follicle destruction. This takes only a few
seconds or less to produce its destructive effect, and after
applying the current there is blanching around the hair follicle and the surrounding area becomes quite red. The hair is
easily pulled out with tweezers, as described above.

There are two ways of employing thermolysis: one technique has a lower intensity of electric current and has to be
maintained for between 3 and 20 seconds. This allows for
slower but longer heating and thus more tissue destruction;
the other technique, known as the *flash technique*, uses a high-
intensity current for a much shorter duration ($\frac{1}{10}$ to $\frac{1}{2}$ of a
second), so that the heat and damage occur rapidly. The
advantages of the flash technique are that as it is so fast, the
client hardly has a chance for any pain to register. Both techniques are frequently used in salons today.

Which method of electrolysis is more effective, galvanic
electrolysis or thermolysis? Some clinicians have found (after
years of experience using both types) that the thermolysis technique is less likely than the galvanic technique to destroy the

hair bulb if the follicle is large, distorted or curled: i.e. the galvanic method is more effective for difficult hairs. They have also found that flash thermolysis is less effective than the slower type, and thus only really useful for fine, straight hairs. However, the one study that has been carried out comparing the two types of electrolysis found no difference in regrowth rates, but only that some of the regrowth hairs treated with thermolysis were smaller in diameter and more likely to be distorted than those treated with galvanic electrolysis. I personally am more inclined to believe the years of experience of several clinicians than one experiment conducted over 20 weeks.

'THE BLEND'

The most recent development, and this may be a solution to the question asked above, has been to combine galvanic electrolysis with thermolysis in a technique called 'the blend'. This means that the hair follicle is subjected to both chemical (more effective) and thermal (more rapid) damage, so that the net effect is a surer and faster method of destruction. It takes a few seconds for the needle to discharge the necessary current. Different clinicians who have tried all three types of electrolysis believe that the blend method is the best available, but proper studies comparing them have not been done. Intuitively, it would seem that this is the best technique, but although becoming more popular, it is still not most frequently used because these machines are much more expensive than the other types.

Commencing Electrolysis

If you have decided to have electrolysis as a way of permanently removing your hair, or you have been referred to an electrologist by your GP, below are brief descriptions of

where you can have it done, the machine used, and what to
expect from the electrologist.

THE SALON

There are several places you as the client might go for electrolysis treatment:

* A private practice
  Most electrolysis salons are privately run, usually in
  combination with a beauty salon but sometimes with a
  hairdressing salon. The salon is usually operated from
  business premises, but can also be run from the
  electrologist's home or can be a mobile service (where she
  visits you at your home).
* An electrology clinic chain
  There are a few large companies that have their
  electrology clinics all over the country; some are even
  international.
* Department store beauty salon
  A lot of large department stores have beauty salons on the
  premises, and these usually offer an electrolysis service.
  The salon can either be privately run or be a branch of the
  electrology chains.
* Hospital electrolysis service
  Some hospitals have this as part of the services offered by
  the dermatology department. All referrals are made by
  hospital doctors, and the service is usually only part-time,
  a few hours once or twice a week.

THE EPILATION MACHINE

There are many different epilation machines on the market.
They differ in price, the type of electrolysis and the range of
current intensity as well as in other ways. There has not been
a controlled study on the effectiveness of different machines.

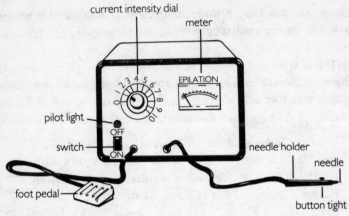

Figure 13: *An epilation machine*

The basic function of these machines is to transmit a regulated and controlled electric current through a lead that has a needle attached at one end (see Figure 13).

The intensity of the current that reaches the needle and the amount of time this current discharges through the needle can be modified and controlled by the operator. The intensity is set by positioning a dial (or equivalent) on the epilation machine; the time the current passes depends on how long the electrologist presses a switch, either on the needle holder or by means of a foot pedal. New epilation machines are now computerized and emit a very accurate level of current. The type of needle used can vary in what it is made of (usually it is stainless steel, but can also be gold or platinum alloys), its length, its thickness (usually a thicker needle is used for a bigger follicle), and whether it has an insulated shaft or not.

The Amount of Current Used

The amount of electric current that enters the skin is a product of the amount of time the current is being administered and the intensity of that current. Both these factors are controlled by the electrologist.

The aim of electrolysis is to introduce enough current into the hair follicle to destroy the hair bulb and cause minimum damage at the skin surface. The higher the intensity of the current and the longer the needle is discharging this current, the more damage will be caused both at the bulb and the skin surface.

As you can imagine, to destroy a thick coarse hair from a large follicle will need a larger amount of electric current than a fine hair in a smaller follicle. Similarly, thick, tough skin will be able to tolerate larger currents better than fine, sensitive skin.

It is up to the electrologist to decide the intensity and duration of current that you need and can tolerate, by assessing your hair growth and your skin type. Some computerized machines calculate the duration of the current once the intensity has been set. Different people tolerate different intensity levels depending upon their skin type and also their threshold of pain. If you can tolerate only a low intensity, then the course of electrolysis to remove your hair permanently will take longer to complete, because hair follicles are likely only to be damaged, and not destroyed, after the first treatment, resulting in a higher regrowth rate (see page 103).

THE ELECTROLOGIST
The electrologist is either a beautician trained in beauty treatments and electrolysis, or someone who is trained only to perform electrolysis. The training is given in either a privately-run school or one of the government education technical colleges. Major cosmetic companies may also sponsor and offer training to individuals.

In the UK an electrologist needs qualifications before she

has the right to work; these qualifications include both practical and theoretical knowledge in the techniques of electrolysis. There are several professional bodies that run courses and give awards, and which are recognized as offering good electrology training (see below).

The length of training varies from six months to two years. The training involves at least 200 hours of practical work and about 40 hours of theory.

Below is a list of recognized diplomas and certificates:

Diploma of Remedial Epilation (DRE)
City & Guilds Beauty Therapist's Certificate 761
City & Guilds Certificate in Electrical Epilation 761–3
The International Beauty Therapist's Diploma
The International CIDESCO Diploma
The Estheticienne Diploma
The Certificate in Epilation
Electrolysis Diploma Course
Beauty Therapy Diploma
Estheticienne Diploma

In your first visit, the electrologist will discuss with you your hair problem and what methods you have used in the past to remove the hair and for how long. She will probably talk about the physiology of hair growth and follicles and discuss how electrolysis works. An explanation of side-effects, regrowth, skin sensitivity and current used should also be given. She will give you an idea of how long appointments will be, how spaced out they should be and may be able to suggest how long the entire process of electrolysis will take for your area of hair.

She will spend time discussing your medical records: electrolysis is contraindicated with certain illnesses (see page 120), and she will want to know if you suffer from any of these. Certain drugs cause growth of body hair, and she should know about these (see page 41). The oral contraceptive pill and certain hormone therapies may also affect hair growth. She will ask about allergies you have, and lastly, the electrologist should know if you have seen your GP about your problem of hair growth. A good electrologist should be able to recognize when a woman should see her GP about the possibility of an underlying hormonal or other problem, although electrologists are not under any obligation to do so, and may in fact be unable to. I believe it is much safer for a woman initially to approach her GP if she is at all worried about her hair growth or related problems, rather than to approach an electrologist or beautician.

The electrologist will inspect the area for electrolysis, and in doing so will have a better idea of how long it might take for complete permanent removal of the hair, bearing in mind difficulties such as skin sensitivity, stubbornness of growth, poor healing, etc.

A discussion about temporary removal of the area of hair while having electrolysis will be necessary, especially if the area of hair is large and embarrassing to the client. I have already mentioned the importance of shaving while undergoing electrolysis (pages 61 and 108) and will stress it again here. Shaving does not increase or thicken hair growth, nor does it distort the follicles. More importantly, it allows the electrologist to work only on growing hairs, which are the only ones successfully electrolysed. If your electrologist says you should not shave, despite your telling her the reasons why shaving is a good idea, I really think you should pack your bags and go. You might waste a lot of money and time if you stay.

Next, she will prepare you for electrolysis: your skin will be cleaned with an antiseptic lotion or a soothing cream, and your make-up will be removed. After preparing the needle and correctly adjusting the dials on the epilation machine she will position herself and will then start electrolysing as I have already described. The effect of the needle and current will be assessed (i.e. the intensity of any pain you experience, your skin's reaction and whether the hairs come out easily), and the current will be modified accordingly (she will change either the intensity or the duration of the current) before the next hair is electrolysed. She will eventually find the current intensity and duration of discharge which will have a minimal effect on your skin surface and yet allow your hairs to come out with no resistance. She will continue to electrolyse hairs in this way until your session is over. Do not be disappointed if the area looks as hairy before the treatment as after. It takes time to clear an area completely.

Afterwards the electrologist will put either a soothing lotion or weak alcohol over the area. You should then discuss frequency of visits, cost, duration of each session and an estimate of how long the whole process will take, as well as any other concerns you might have about electrolysis.

The Effectiveness of Electrolysis

Electrolysis is a very expensive and time-consuming activity. For these and other reasons it is essential to maximize its effectiveness so that women can be permanently hair-free as quickly and as cheaply as possible, thereby reducing the number of women who give up because of its ineffectiveness or expense. Sadly, women who turn to electrolysis as the only hope for a permanent treatment are rarely told by their GP or the electrologist how to make the most of this process, and as a result hundreds of pounds and hundreds of hours are wasted, just because certain guidelines are not laid out (see below).

There are two factors that determine the effectiveness of electrolysis:

1. Side-effects
   The numbers and severity of side-effects have to be considered acceptable by women if electrolysis is to be regarded as a successful procedure. They will be discussed later in this chapter.
2. Rate of regrowth
   Regrowth is defined as the growth of a new hair from a follicle which has previously been electrolysed. A perfectly treated hair follicle under ideal conditions will not regrow a hair after one treatment of electrolysis. However, reality is not so perfect. Even with a good electrologist under ideal conditions a client will still get regrowth rates of between 20 and 40 per cent, i.e. about ⅓ of the hair follicles electrolysed will grow a new hair and need another treatment of electrolysis.

There are probably many reasons why regrowth occurs in spite of what seem to be good working conditions, but the two main ones are human error and body physiology, and I would imagine that even with extra precautions a regrowth of less than 10 to 20 per cent would be difficult to obtain. (You can compare this to dusting your house; there will always be some little areas that you missed, others that were not visible, and still others which were difficult to reach and do properly, so that even with careful dusting, the house is never 100 per cent free of dust).

However, there is no doubt that a significant number of women have experienced regrowth rates much higher than this, and some women have really not benefited at all from electrolysis. What usually happens in these cases is that the woman has electrolysis for what seems like a very long time, yet her hair growth does not appear to be reducing. She becomes disillusioned, and either stops the treatment and goes back to temporary methods of removal, or continues

with the electrolysis in spite of the fact that the area of hair
does not become sparser and her visits to the electrologist do
not become less frequent. These cases are not what electrolysis
should be; there is *always* an underlying reason for this high
regrowth rate; reason, or reasons, which can be found and
stopped.

Below I have described the main factors that lead to an
increase in the regrowth rate after electrolysis:

CAUSES OF HIGH REGROWTH RATE

1. Underlying Hormonal Imbalance

A woman is more likely to approach a beauty salon rather
than her GP to get help for excess body hair. In the majority
of cases there will be no underlying hormonal abnormality,
and the electrolysis will be successful. However, if there is a
hormonal imbalance then electrolysis has a reduced effectiveness, and in some cases is barely effective at all for permanent hair removal.

As I have already described, the hormonal imbalance is most
likely to be due to an excess of the male hormones called *androgens* (see page 33). The effect of androgens on the hair follicle
is to increase the thickness and speed of growth of the hair,
and also to stimulate dormant hair follicles into action. This
means that hair follicles are made larger by androgens, and will
therefore need more current and time to destroy them. These
follicles are thus more likely to produce regrowth hairs. But
more importantly, since about 20 per cent of hair follicles are
dormant under normal hormonal levels, these, in the presence
of excess androgen, will begin to grow hairs.

As one researcher described, to clear an area of ground, it
is not enough to pull out the weeds, you also have to prepare
the soil. Likewise, electrolysis may be able temporarily to
remove the area of hairs, but if there is an underlying excess

of androgens new follicles will continue to be activated, small follicles will grow larger, and hair growth overall may not lessen. What is needed in these cases is anti-androgenic medication to reduce the levels of androgens in the blood and thus stop their persisting effects on hair growth.

The electrologist may be alerted to this possibility at the initial consultation, but if not then she should realize when it becomes evident that the electrolysis is not working. It is not clear to me whose responsibility it is to recognize that there may be some underlying hormonal problem. Certainly, electrologists are taught basic medical reasons for ineffective electrolysis, and they should have some idea of how quickly to expect a particular area of hair to be permanently cleared. However, a client should also try to be aware of what is happening, although I realize that this is not as easy as it may sound. If an underlying hormonal imbalance is in the slightest way suspected, the client should see her GP for tests and an examination.

2. The Resting Phase of the Hair Follicle is Not Amenable to Electrolysis

I have already described the different phases of growth of a hair and its follicle in Chapter 2. Understanding and applying this knowledge is essential in order to reduce hours of unnecessary electrolysis.

There are three phases of the growth cycle of a hair (see also Figure 14):

1. Growth phase: when the hair is actively growing and the germinating cells and the hair bulb are both deep and continuous with the hair shaft.
2. Resting phase: when the hair is resting, the 'club bulb' is shallow, but the germinating cells are deep.
3. Intermediate phase: the very brief transitional phase between these two.

The hair can also be in a dormant phase. This occurs after a hair has fallen out (i.e. the end of the resting phase), and instead of a new hair growing back quickly, the follicle remains dormant and can stay in this state for weeks to years. About 20 per cent of hair follicles are dormant.

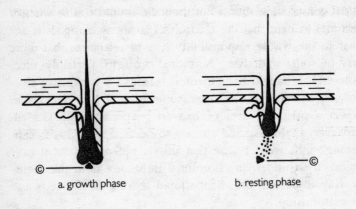

a. growth phase　　　　　　　　b. resting phase

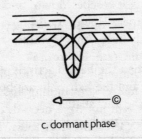

c. dormant phase

Figure 14: Positions of germinating cells at different phases of the growth cycle

What is the effect of electrolysis on each of these phases?

In the growth phase, since the germinating cells (i.e. those cells that give the hair follicle the potential for growing a hair) are at the bottom of the hair bulb, it is easy for the electrolysis needle to reach down and discharge current around them. Thus electrolysis will be effective in almost all cases as long as a sufficient amount of current is discharged (see Figure 15).

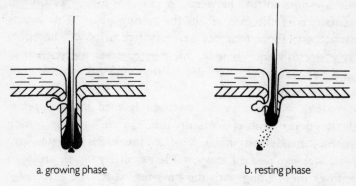

a. growing phase   b. resting phase

Figure 15: *Position of electrolysis needle during different phases of the growth cycle*

In the resting phase, the end of the follicle will be at the bottom of the club bulb, and this is where the needle will naturally feel resistance as it reaches down, and it will be unable to penetrate any deeper. However, the germinating cells are deeper than the club bulb, and therefore these will not be reached by the needle (see Figure 15). So, when a resting hair is electrolysed, although the hair might come out easily because its attachments to surrounding tissue are destroyed, the germinating cells will not have been disturbed and a new hair will *always* grow. It is therefore *useless* for a hair in the resting phase to be electrolysed, it might as well have been plucked for all the good it will do.

The intermediate phase is so short and infrequent that it hardly ever gets electrolysed, while the dormant hair follicle has no hair to electrolyse in the first place.

The next factor to consider is how many hairs are in each phase of the cycle at any given time.

If only a few hairs are in the resting phase, then there is no point making a fuss about them, but if there are many, then it is worth taking this into consideration.

It is estimated that between 15 per cent to 50 per cent of the hairs over the face are in the resting phase. This means that at best, about four out of every five hairs will be effectively electrolysed – at worst, only every other hair will be effectively electrolysed. You would basically be throwing half your money and time away.

For hair on the legs the situation is even more extreme. About 70 per cent of hairs on the legs are in their resting phase – that is just under ¾ of all the hairs. For this area then, ¾ of your time and money will be wasted if your electrologist removes these along with the growing hairs. The percentage of resting hairs in other areas of the body probably fall somewhere between these two figures.

I think these figures should convince you that it is definitely worth your time and money to electrolyse only growing hairs and to leave resting hairs alone, letting them fall out naturally and allowing them to start their own growing phase later.

The last question addresses how one can distinguish between resting and growing hairs.

It is easy: all you have to do is shave. By shaving, you cut all hairs to the level of the skin. Only those in their growing phase will continue to grow. Those in their resting phase will stay at the level of the skin. The electrologist therefore has a sample of only growing hairs from which to choose. If you shave one to three days before having electrolysis (and the exact number of days needed can be discussed beforehand with your electrologist) there should be enough of the growing shafts visible for them to be removed.

This method of shaving while having electrolysis treatment is common practice in a lot of clinics in North America, but in the UK women are still actively discouraged from shaving. *If you cannot convince your electrologist of the benefits of shaving, try showing her this book — or find yourself another electrologist.*

3. Distorted Roots and Follicle

The process of electrolysis, wherein the needle is inserted into the follicle, is a 'blind' procedure, because it all happens under the skin. The electrologist must sense whether the needle is in the right place, and this comes with practice. Most often, the hair follicle is directly below the hair shaft, and so it is not difficult to guide the needle correctly. However, sometimes the follicle is distorted, and in this case it will be very difficult to get to the base of it with the needle. In a similar way, certain skin and hair types are more likely to have curled follicles (black skin, for example; see Figure 16), making the process of electrolysis more difficult.

These follicles have a high regrowth rate after electrolysis, because the germinating cells are frequently not electrolysed enough to destroy them (because of their difficult positioning). It takes an experienced electrologist to deal with them, and it might be worth using either the blend technique or galvanized electrolysis, both of which have been reported to be the more effective methods of electrolysis for these follicles.

Although no proper studies have been done, it is often quoted that waxing or plucking distorts the follicle, and certainly an experienced electrologist can tell if an area of hair has been previously treated with such methods of temporary hair removal, because the roots are different from those of untreated hair. It is therefore advisable that you do not use these methods of hair removal while undergoing electrolysis, because you are likely to distort follicles even more and make the electrolysis more difficult and time-consuming.

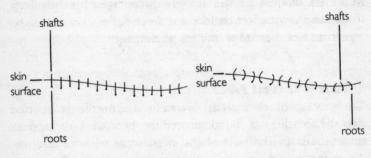

a. Mongolian skin and hair   b. Black skin and hair

Figure 16: The follicles of Mongolian and black skin

4. Client on Certain Medication

Certain drugs have the unwanted side-effect of causing excess body hair – these have been discussed fully on page 41. Before starting electrolysis, the first consultation should include asking about any drugs the client is taking. If the electrologist is not sure if a particular drug promotes the growth of body hair, the client should be referred to his or her GP to confirm its effect (there are many men who under-go electrolysis, to remove for instance excess hair on their shoulders, between their eyebrows or in tandem with a sex change).

The drugs are of two types: they either cause growth of hair in the 'male pattern' (i.e. hirsutism) – these drugs are related to androgens and their effects – or they cause hair growth over the whole body (i.e. hypertrichosis) – these probably act in a variety of ways (see page 41).

If the client is on medication which causes either hirsutism or hypertrichosis, it can often be substituted for another drug that does not cause this side-effect. This hair growth may be fully reversible once the drug has stopped, or it may become reduced with stopping the drug. In some cases, sadly, hair growth is not reversible, and even after stopping the drug continues as strongly as before.

Before electrolysis is started the client should have an understanding of the effect of the drug while on it, what happens once she has stopped it, and whether it can be replaced by another type of drug. For example, if the drug can be stopped and the hair growth is completely reversible, electrolysis will not be necessary. Or if stopping the drug reduces hair growth, the client might want to wait and see this reduction before embarking on the expense of electrolysis.

5. The Electrologist

There is no doubt that there are some electrologists who are excellent and others who are not, while the majority lie somewhere between. It is interesting that being a good electrologist appears to have little to do with the degree of training and more to do with an intrinsic skill and concern: some newly-qualified electrologists are better than ones who have been working for years. Since they are not going to tell you if they are not any good, it is up to you to find out. There are a couple of pointers which might suggest that a particular electrologist is not good at electrolysing.

1. I have mentioned that once a hair has had enough electric current applied to it, its attachments to the surrounding tissues will loosen and the hair can be pulled out of its follicle (by plucking) without resistance. The electrologist should be aware of resistance to plucking; and if there is

any, she should not pluck out the hair but rather consider what went wrong, and then re-treat the hair.
2. You should look out for the levels of hygiene and care that she applies to your skin and hair. A sloppy worker is more likely to be a sloppy electrologist.

What kind of things could she do wrong?

6. Probing Incorrectly
Directing the needle correctly can only be done with careful probing and insertion. The needle can be inserted too shallowly, too deeply, into the sebaceous gland, into the wall of the follicle, or just not into the follicle at all (see Figure 17).

If the electrologist is working either carelessly or at incredible speed, without appearing to be carefully selective about where she places the needle, it is more likely than not that the needle will be badly placed. Imagine, she has to insert the needle into a tiny opening, then has to gently push it along the length of the hidden hair, and then, when she feels resistance upon reaching the bottom of the follicle, she must stop and apply the current.

If you have someone electrolysing at a very fast rate it is unlikely that the care needed to remove a hair permanently is being given. Ideally, you want to find an electrologist who takes time over each hair from the moment of inserting the needle to when she gently pulls out the hair. If the hair does not come out with minimal pulling, then she should reinsert the needle and re-treat the hair with another dose of current. If she regularly pulls out hairs that seem to be well attached, you are effectively paying for a plucking session and not an electrolysis session. Far better to have your electrologist remove 30 hairs per session permanently than 100 temporarily.

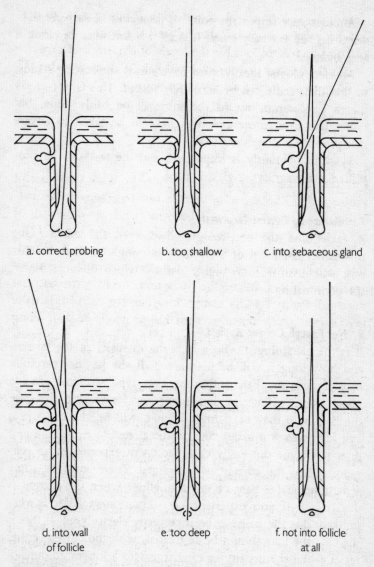

a. correct probing

b. too shallow

c. into sebaceous gland

d. into wall
of follicle

e. too deep

f. not into follicle
at all

Figure 17: Probing

Another very important point: If the insertion of the needle hurts, then it has been incorrectly placed. It should only hurt when the current is being discharged.

An electrologist ideally must have steady, unshaking hands, so that the needle can be accurately placed. This is not to say that a fine tremor means the job will be badly done, but rather that even more care will have to be taken to ensure that probing is done correctly.

Eyesight obviously is important, and the task can be simplified if a magnifying glass is used.

7. Discharging Current Incorrectly

If each time the electrologist discharges the current she moves her hand out of the follicle just slightly, then the current will dissipate into higher tissues, which do not contain the germinating cells.

8. Not Enough Current Applied

It is the electrologist who selects the intensity of the current and how long it will be discharged. If she has not carefully considered your hair and your skin type she may decide upon a level of current that is too low for you. In this case the hair bulb may be damaged but it will not be destroyed, and regrowth will occur. She can be alerted to this if the hair does not come out easily or if the client experiences no sensation when the current is discharged. There must be some sensation felt (of pain or just a tingling) when the current is discharged. If you experience no sensation at all it is very unlikely that the hair has been correctly electrolysed. If this is the case the hair should be re-treated, with the current either set at a higher intensity or discharged for a longer amount of time.

Initial Temporary Clearance of Hair

One frequent disappointment women have with electrolysis is that it seems that the same hair follicles continue to grow new hairs despite multiple electrolysis treatments. They find that each time they have a session of electrolysis, the hairs are successfully cleared from the skin, but within a few weeks it looks as though they have all grown back. This is not necessarily a problem of excess regrowth, as described above, but rather the appearance of hairs that were previously below the skin surface.

You have to remember that the number of hair follicles that are successfully electrolysed at any one session is only a fraction of the total number of follicles that have to be electrolysed eventually. So at each electrolysis session new and different follicles are being treated (plus the 20 per cent of previously treated follicles that have regrowth hairs).

What do I mean by this? Let us take the face as an example.

Over the face about ⅓ of the hairs are resting (i.e. not growing), about ½ of the hairs are growing, about ⅙ of the hair follicles are dormant (i.e. there is no hair in these follicles), and a tiny fraction of hairs are in the process of changing from growing to resting. Let us suppose that you are shaving your face, so that only the growing hairs are seen by the electrologist. Of the hairs that are growing, some will be under the skin surface slowly making their way up and will therefore be invisible to the electrologist. This means that at the first electrolysis session the electrologist has less than ⅓ of all the follicles to work with and destroy. Even if she clears this area completely over a period of a few weeks, with each new session a few of the resting hairs will have entered the growing phase, a few of the hairs growing under the skin will now be protruding, and at least 20 per cent of the follicles previously electrolysed will begin to produce a regrowth hair. And I have not yet mentioned the follicles that are dormant, about ⅛th of the total, that have the potential to start growing a hair at any time.

Lastly, there are some follicles that have more than one hair growing from them. These are called *multiple follicular hair units* (see Figure 18), and have only one opening to the skin but two or more hairs protruding from this opening with two or more follicles underneath. This means that there are several follicles which need to be treated with electrolysis from a single opening.

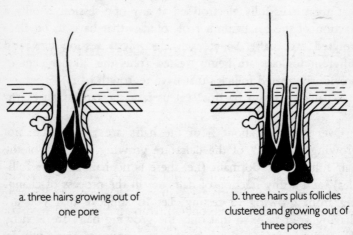

a. three hairs growing out of
one pore

b. three hairs plus follicles
clustered and growing out of
three pores

Figure 18: Multiple follicular hair units

So you can see that what you might consider unsuccessful electrolysis is in fact the initial process of temporary clearance that every area of hair has to go through before permanent clearance is achieved. So do not be disillusioned. If you are not shaving the area of hair, however, then the problem is much greater: another 30 per cent of your hairs will later regrow (making a total of 50 per cent regrowth) because they were electrolysed during a time when the germinating cells could not be reached by the current, i.e. they were effectively only plucked out.

So three very important messages:

1. If you can shave an area while having electrolysis, it is well worth it to do so.
2. Do not be disillusioned if initially you think that the electrolysis is not working; it is likely that for the valid reasons described above changes are initially slow.
3. It is very important to try and recognize when electrolysis really is not working, to understand why this is, and to act upon it.

Estimation of Time and Cost for Specific Areas of Hair

COST

Electrolysis is not cheap, although costs vary somewhat from salon to salon.

Some countries have private medical insurance that will cover the cost of electrolysis. In Canada, some forms of medical insurance will pay if excess hair is caused by higher-than-normal levels of testosterone[2]. In America, medical insurance will not pay for electrolysis despite a woman having high levels of testosterone. In Britain, private health insurance might pay, but only if the psychological stress caused by the

---

[2] Specifically, if the level of testosterone, free testosterone or DHEA-S is 25 per cent above the stated laboratory maximum (in women 30 or younger). For women over 30 years of age, the DHEA-S must be double normal (while testosterone and free testosterone must be 25 per cent above normal).

excess hair is judged to be immense (they would need a covering letter from a Consultant). Regarding drug-induced hair growth, some forms of Canadian insurance will pay for electrolysis[3] – it might be worth inquiring about this wherever you are living. If you have private insurance, no matter where you live, it might also be worth inquiring about.

Normally, you can book electrolysis for 5-, 10-, 15-, 20-, 30-, 45- or 60-minute sessions, and sometimes for even longer. The longer the electrolysis time, the cheaper it is per minute, so it is worth trying to have less frequent but longer visits (if your skin can take it). It is not worth me writing down costs of sessions, because by the time you are reading this book the figures will be out of date. You can phone your local beauty clinic and ask how much each session costs; I am sure they will be happy to oblige.

TIME

It is impossible to give very accurate estimates of how long you will need electrolysis to permanently clear an area of hair, because each client is different in the many factors that affect hair growth and the ability to be electrolysed optimally, for example: age, pain threshold, skin sensitivity to the current, coarseness of hair, distortion of follicles, number of coarse hairs, cause of hair growth, underlying hormone state, etc. However, a rough estimate can be given for average situations and areas of hair[4].

- Post-menopausal facial hair growth
  The average post-menopausal woman with a number of coarse hairs that have been growing for the past few years

---

[3] Caused by androgenic hormones, Dilantin, cyclosporin, high-dose long-term cortisone and danazol.

[4] These figures are taken from estimates from two sources (see references).

or so over her upper lip, sides of her mouth and chin:

Initially, weekly-to-biweekly visits of 20 to 30 minutes in length over 2 to 4 months.

Then, biweekly-to-monthly visits of 10 to 20 minutes for 2 to 4 months.

Lastly, 1 to 2 visits each year to remove the new hairs that will continue to grow from other follicles (this is not regrowth, but rather the continuing process of getting hairier over the face after the menopause).

- Average young female with moustache
  This is a common area for epilation in young woman; and on average there is a distinct area of hair from the centre of the moustache area down to beyond the edges of the lip:

  Initially, weekly visits of 15 to 30 minutes for 6 to 9 months.

  Then, biweekly-to-monthly visits of 15 to 30 minutes for 6 to 9 months.

  Lastly, maintenance would be 1 to 2 visits each year for several years.

- Woman with marked facial hair growth
  A woman who needs to shave every day because of excessive, coarse hair growth, which can encompass areas as extensive as the moustache, chin, sideburns, cheeks and neck:

  Initially, 3 hours each week for about a year.

  Then, 1 hour each week for a year.

  By this time hair growth has diminished considerably, however the time taken to maintain this state of reducing hair growth down to no hair growth varies markedly with different women.

- The beard growth of transsexuals
  Initially, 1 hour a week for 2+ years.

  Then, 30 minutes a week for 6 months.

Lastly, maintenance would be 1 to 2 visits each year for a few years.
- Nipple hair
  A few hairs on the nipples will take a total of between 1 and 5 hours of electrolysis to be permanently removed.
- Underarm hair
  In an average person it takes about 10 hours to clear these hairs permanently.
- Arm and leg hair
  Obviously, the size of this area varies markedly from person to person, as do the growth and type of hair, thus it is very difficult (if not impossible) to give average times for permanent hair removal. However, one of the references I used suggested that the amount of time necessary in order to clear this hair is similar to that needed for the thick facial hair growth.

Contraindications to Electrolysis

There are several medical conditions which should be considered before embarking on a course of electrolysis; however, absolute contraindications are very rare. The more likely scenario is that an electrologist does not want to treat a client with a particular underlying illness because of her fear that something might happen to the client during the procedure or afterwards.

PACEMAKERS
Certain pacemakers are affected by the passage of electric current through the body. Thus all clients with pacemakers need to get permission from their cardiologist before starting electrolysis.

HEART CONDITIONS

Any person with a 'weak' heart (e.g. angina, previous heart attacks, heart failure) is more susceptible to stress and anxiety, but this does not mean that these people lead stress- and anxiety-free lives. They should be aware of their own limitations, and pace themselves accordingly, both in everyday life and when undergoing electrolysis.

EPILEPSY

An epileptic attack can be triggered by a number of things, including stress and one's psychological, emotional or physical state. Just as frequently these attacks come without warning and with no apparent trigger. Someone whose condition is well controlled by medication may not have an attack for years, while others, despite regular high-dose medication, may get attacks monthly to yearly.

Electrolysis as an electrical procedure is unlikely to initiate an attack, however electrolysis as an anticipated stressful and painful procedure may affect the client's well-being, which could, as with any stressful event, precipitate an attack. Lastly, since an epileptic attack is as likely to occur at home as in the street or in the salon, there is a risk that a client could have one while undergoing electrolysis. I am sure that most electrologists would want the permission of their client's GP before agreeing to undertake electrolysis, but the final decision whether to go ahead or not usually lies with the electrologist herself and whether she wants to take responsibility for treating such a client considering the risks involved.

DIABETES

The problem with diabetics is that their skin is more susceptible to infections and heals slowly once an infection has established itself. So again, an electrologist would probably want permission from the client's GP before initiating electrolysis.

These clients will also need to be extra careful with their skin hygiene before and after each electrolysis session.

ASTHMA
Asthma sufferers have attacks which are precipitated either by specific external causes (e.g. a cold or specific allergens like cat hair) or by less specific internal events (such as stress or anxiety). An asthma sufferer can have only very mild attacks or life-threatening ones, and they can occur frequently (monthly) or very rarely (every few years). An asthma sufferer can be on regular high-dose medication to prevent frequent or life-threatening attacks, or she can take medication only when she feels an attack might be starting or to prevent an attack in certain situations (for example, before taking exercise).

It would be wise for the electrologist to know what kind of asthma the client has, so as to be aware of a possible attack, but ultimately the asthmatic looks after herself as much at the dentist as in a beauty salon, and only expects common sense from those people that happen to be around.

ACNE, BACTERIAL AND VIRAL SKIN INFECTIONS
The ideal situation is for the client to suffer no skin infections, so that there is no risk of re-infecting other skin sites. There is a documented case of flat warts (which are viral infections) being spread by the electrolysis needle, and the inoculation of the herpes virus (the cold sore) is not difficult to imagine. Likewise a client with badly-controlled acne is more susceptible to re-infection, as are those patients with other bacterial infections (e.g. impetigo).

Ideally an electrologist should not put her needle through any of the above-mentioned lesions on the skin surface. However, there is a difficulty associated with acne. Commonly, women who suffer from moderate to severe hirsutism also suffer from acne, and they should not be denied electrolysis just because of the presence of these spots. As long as their acne is fairly well controlled (and nowadays there are excellent topical and oral treatments), and a test of electrolysis reveals no apparent ill-effects, then it can be undertaken and continued. The other problem that arises with acne sufferers is hyperpigmentation at each needle site.

What happens is that the pores are often impregnated with sebum and melanin pigment (the blackness from a black-head is not dirt, but melanin). If such a pore is electrolysed there is a possibility of impregnating this melanin deeper into the skin tissue, leaving a permanent dark mark (rather than the melanin being simply in the follicle as in a blackhead, which can be removed by squeezing it). This is called *tattooing*, and occurs whenever a dark particle is pushed into an area of skin where it should not be (like coal miners who develop tattoo-like markings over their hands and other areas).

BACTERIAL ENDOCARDITIS AND INFECTION OF PROSTHETIC DEVICES

Any one with a heart valve lesion, or with an artificial pros-thesis (for example an artificial heart valve, hip joint, knee joint, etc.) is at risk of infection at this site if certain bacteria enter their bloodstream from the outside and settle down and multiply there. There has been one documented case of someone developing a particular endocarditis (infection around the heart valves) after electrolysis. Some cardiologists believe that the slightest external infection (for example infected eczema) should be treated with antibiotics so that bacteria are unable to multiply in the blood. Others believe that only more infective procedures (for example having dental treatment) should be treated with antibiotics. If you have any of the above conditions it is worth consulting your GP to ask his or her advice.

SKIN PRONE TO SCARRING, HYPERPIGMENTATION, OR HYPOPIGMENTATION

Certain skins are more affected by trauma than others. For example, some skins form raised scars with trauma (called keloid scars), others develop more pigmentation in the area (hyperpigmentation), still others less pigmentation (hypo-pigmentation). Whether electrolysis will have this effect can only be found out by testing a small area and seeing what happens. It is very rare that electrolysis does cause any of these problems. Sadly, it is more likely that these kinds of blemishes (especially over the face) were caused by previous plucking (see page 71). A client should not be put off electrolysis because she scars easily, at least not before the electrologist has tried electrolysing a small area of her skin.

Problems and Side-effects

It seems that most people do not experience many problems with electrolysis, and the problems that are frequently experienced are mild ones.

PAIN

Some women feel a fair degree of pain while having electrolysis, and for a very small minority this pain is so great that it prevents them from continuing treatment. The obvious way of minimizing the pain is to put yourself in the right psychological frame of mind by consciously breathing and concentrating on something other than the electrolysis. An alternative quick-fix method of reducing the pain is to take an aspirin or similar painkiller half an hour to an hour before the appointment. In one clinic in Canada, ice is provided on the premises to apply to the area five to ten minutes before the treatment, which helps deaden the area to sensation. This same clinic has also tried applying creams that were advertised as being able to reduce pain, but these did not worked. It may be some relief to know that after a few treatments the pain seems to lessen.

REDNESS AND FOLLICULITIS

After treatment, almost all people will experience some degree of redness around the area, and some will also suffer folliculitis (where the area around each follicle is raised and red). This is the reaction of your skin to the tissue damage occurring to each follicle. It can be reduced by taking an aspirin half an hour to an hour beforehand (paracetamol will not help because it has no anti-inflammatory properties). After the electrolysis you could try a natural soothing agent (for example wych-hazel, elderflower water or calamine lotion), or a light non-perfumed moisturizer. Something more medical such as a topical antihistamine (for example caladryl) is also worth trying.

If the reaction is really quite bad, applying a very mild hydrocortisone cream over the area works very well. Strengths of 0.5 per cent and 1 per cent hydrocortisone cream can be bought over the counter (they are available over the counter, which should give you some indication of how very safe they are). If they are used as indicated they have no side-effects even after a few years of intermittent use. (I am aware of the steroid-phobia among the general public, but the creams I have mentioned do not belong in this category). Try the weaker one first, and if this does not help, go on to the 1 per cent. It should be applied sparingly, but you should still find it very effective. This redness and folliculitis should resolve within four to eight hours.

CRUSTING, SCABBING AND SWELLING

A small amount of scabbing just around the follicles is not uncommon, and is caused by the electric current spreading upwards to the skin surface. It can be reduced by decreasing the current's intensity or duration, however sometimes this reduced level of current will not be enough to detach the hair; in these cases some scabbing is inevitable. It will heal completely, and usually does so within two to four days.

A great deal of scabbing and crusting and some swelling can occur if the current is much too high or if the skin is very sensitive. Again, it will heal quickly, and at your next appointment a lower current will be used. If you are so sensitive that even low currents have this effect, then it is up to you to decide whether you want to continue treatment and suffer scabs for several days after each session or give the treatment up.

HYPERPIGMENTATION AND HYPOPIGMENTATION

Some people develop excess pigmentation at sites of trauma, and less frequently others develop a reduction of pigmentation in the skin after trauma. Electrolysis is sometimes enough to induce either of these effects. Occasionally small amounts of brown pigmentation develop over the upper lip, but these usually disappear within months (do not confuse this with the appearance of a distinct brown line, just above your lip and along it. This is not caused by electrolysis but by the oral contraceptive pill, and is usually irreversible).

Other causes of pigmentation are excessive acne (see page 124) and also occasionally the galvanized electrolysis method or the inadvertent mis-connection of the leads. What happens is that metal molecules leave the needle and enter your skin, causing an indelible mark. This, however, is very rare nowadays. If you are developing hyperpigmentation, I would try to reduce your response to trauma by taking an aspirin beforehand — or even better try hydrocortisone cream afterwards. If this does not help try a reduced current, or maybe change to a different electrologist who uses a different machine.

SCARRING

If electrolysis is done correctly on normal skin there should be no scarring. One clinician with 135,000 hours of electrolysis experience saw scarring only once, and this was very fine pitted scarring on sensitive skin. The other causes of scarring are:

- very sensitive skin which is unable to take the trauma of electrolysis,
- skin which scars easily (i.e. those people prone to keloid scars), and
- deep infection in the follicle following electrolysis (in people who are prone to infection or who don't heal well).

Scarring as a result of any of these causes is very rare. The more common scenario is of someone already scarred by previous treatments (for example plucking) or severe acne, who believes incorrectly that her scarring has been caused by the electrolysis.

INGROWING HAIRS

Just as for any treatment that removes hairs from the root, those hairs that do regrow may potentially develop into ingrowing hairs (see page 83).

Self-electrolysis

ELECTRONIC TWEEZERS

There are several manufacturers that offer home electrolysis devices, in the form of electronic tweezers. Sadly, these devices do not permanently remove hair as claimed, and have not been recognized by the medical profession as resulting in permanent hair removal. The claim is that the current travels down the hair shaft and reaches the bulb, where it is then discharged into the hair bulb and surrounding tissue. What the manufacturers do not tell you is that hair is a very poor conductor of electric current, so that hardly any current reaches the bulb. In America several complaints have been made successfully against these manufacturers, and rightly so. I strongly suggest that you do not waste your money on these devices if you want permanent removal of your hair. They are, however, very effective as plucking devices!

NEEDLE DEVICES

These are battery-operated devices; they use the galvanic method of electrolysis (see page 93). Once the needle is in place it takes ages for enough current to go from the battery to the end of the needle and for the hair to be dislodged (at least a few minutes), but I cannot claim that they do not work. If you had no more than several hairs that you wanted to electrolyse, and you could get very close to them, then this might be an efficient home remedy. However, if you have more hairs and they are positioned so that you cannot see the pore easily (for example, on your face), then I suggest that you do not waste your money.

HOME EPILATION MACHINE

I am sure if someone tried hard enough, she could buy the salon-type of epilation machine without having any training in electrolysis. It is true that if you wanted to electrolyse a very large area of your body then you would probably save a lot of money by purchasing your own machine. However, it really is impossible to see your own tiny pores and the opening on the skin unless your nose and eyes are directly above the area. This means that you could probably successfully electrolyse above your knees and inner calves, but your face (where you would depend upon your reflection to guide you) and your underarm, bikini line, thighs, tummy, etc.

would be practically impossible to do by yourself. If you and a friend wanted to do electrolysis on each other, the idea is more feasible. However, I do cringe at the thought of two pairs of inexperienced hands with an electrolysis machine and a lot of small, hairy follicles. You would be at risk of permanent scarring, pitting, infection and a lot of heartache. If you have not got enough money to pay for electrolysis done properly, I understand the anguish you must feel. But it really is not worth risking permanent damage to your skin.

Electrolysis in the USA and Australia

USA
The laws regarding the right to practise electrolysis in North America are regulated by each individual state. Each state has different regulations, and the diversity of the legal requirements for practise is enormous. Some states require no minimum training before allowing someone to practise as an electrologist, while others require thousands of hours of practice. Some states require an examination of competence, others none. This discrepancy in training and requirements has been the subject of criticism both in the area of medicine and cosmetics, however nothing as yet has changed.

Below is a list of the states and their requirements:

State training	Minimum hours	State exam
Alabama	1,200	yes
Alaska	no state law	no
Arizona	no state law	no
Arkansas	200	yes
California	500	yes
Colorado	no state law	no
Connecticut	120	yes
Delaware	300	yes
District of Columbia	none required	no
Florida	no state law	no
Georgia	no state law	no
Hawaii	600	yes
Idaho	800	yes
Illinois	no state law	no
Indiana	1,200	no
Iowa	100	yes
Kansas	1,100	yes
Kentucky	no state law	no
Louisiana	600	yes
Maine	none required	no
Maryland	100	yes
Massachusetts	1,100	yes
Michigan	300	yes
Minnesota	no state law	no
Mississippi	no state law	no
Missouri	no state law	no
Montana	600	yes
Nebraska	no state law	no
Nevada	1,000	yes
New Hampshire	1,000	no

State training	Minimum hours	State exam
New Jersey	no state law	no
New Mexico	500	yes
New York	no state law	no
North Carolina	no state law	no
North Dakota	300	no
Ohio	500	yes
Oklahoma	600	yes
Oregon	no state law	no
Pennsylvania	no state law	no
Rhode Island	650	yes
South Carolina	no state law	no
South Dakota	2,100	yes
Tennessee	no state law	no
Texas	no state law	no
Utah	500	yes
Vermont	no state law	no
Virginia	no state law	no
Washington	no state law	no
West Virginia	none required	no
Wisconsin	280	yes
Wyoming	no state law	no

AUSTRALIA

There is no governing body or examination in Australia regulating the practice of electrolysis, so basically anyone can start up as an electrologist with little or even no experience. The privately-run courses are usually very short, with only a few days of electrolysis practice. For this reason, a lot of Australian beauticians go to America or Europe for further training, where the courses are much more complete, and they then return to Australia to work. Before you embark on electrolysis in Australia, it would be worth asking about details of the training course your electrologist went through.

References

R. N. Richards and G. E. Meharg, Information and booklets on electrolysis for the patients at the electrolysis clinic in Leslie Street, Toronto, Canada: Willowdale, 1990.

A. Gallent, Principles and Techniques for the Electrologist, Stanley Thornes Publishers Ltd, 1983.

all of references R. B. Greenblatt, V. B. Mahesh, R. D. Gambrell (eds.), The Cause and Management of Hirsutism, Parthenon Publishing, 1987.

INDEX

abdominal hair   32
abrasives   69–70
  pros and cons   69–70
  side-effects   69
acne   41, 45, 122–3
adrenal gland   29
aesthetics   5
anabolic steroids   43
anagen   24–5
androgen   16, 34
  drugs   42–3
anorexia nervosa   40
asexual hair   15
aspirin   79
attitudes, to body hair
  1–12

bleaching,   54–8
  pros and cons   58
  side-effects   56–8
bimanual examination
  45
bulb, hair   19

catagen   25–6
chest hair   32
consultation, medical
  40
cortisone   43
cultural attitudes, to body
  hair   3, 11–12
cyclosporin   43
cyproterone acetate

(Dianette)
  49–50
depilation   58–70
depilatory cream   63–4,
  65–9
  application   67
  pros and cons   68
  side-effects   67–8
  smell   65–6
dermal papilla   19
disguise   53–8
distorted roots   80
dormant follicles   27
drugs   41–4, 110–11
  androgenic 42–3
  cortisone   43
  cyclosporin   43
  Danazol   42–3
  diazoxide   44
  oral contraceptive   42
  penicillamine   44
  phenytoin   43
  to reduce hair   47–50

emotional distress   37
electrolysis   90–132, **92**
  contraindications
  120–4
  cost   117–18
  effectiveness   102–4
  methods   91–6
    blend   96
    galvanic   93–5

    thermolysis   95
  reasons for failure
  104–15
  side-effects   103,
  124–7
  time taken 118–20
epilation   70–89
  electric   73
    pros and cons 73–4,
    74
  threading   75
  waxing   75–89
eyebrows   9–10

facial hair   18, 30
family background   39
fashion   3–4, 6
femininity   1–2
follicles   13, 18–29, **21**,
  34–7
  dormant   27
  sheath   22

germinating cells   19, **21**
glands   31
growth cycle, of hair
  23–7, **24**, **26**
growth phase   23, 24–5
  involution phase   23,
  25–7
  resting phase   23, 27

heat   36

hirsutism 37
historical attitudes 6–8, 10–11
hormones 15, 16–18, 41, 51
hydrocortisone 79–80
hygiene 5
hyperpigmentation 82–3, 124, 126–7
hypertrichosis 38, 43
hypopigmentation 124, 126–7

infected spots 80–1
ingrowing hair 64, 68, 83–9
inherited characteristics 36
involution phase, 23, 25–7

keratin 22

lower back hair 32
lower leg hair 32–3

make-up 58
masculinity 1–2
medical history 40–1
melanin 22
mental illness, effect on body hair 37

natural body hair 3

oestrogen 16
oral contraceptive 42, 48–9

pattern of growth of body hair 40
pelvic scan 46
physical significance of body hair 6
physiological nature of body hair 13–52
pilosebaceous unit 19, 20
plucking 70–3
  side-effects 71–2
polycystic ovarian disease 50
pores 13, 19
pregnancy, effect on body hair 36–7
puberty 29–30
pubic hair 8–9

racial groups 35–7
razors 62–4
  electric 62
  safety 62–4
  side-effects 62–4
red hair 54–5
resting phase 23, 105–9
ritual and religion 5
root 19

scarring, by electrolysis 127
sebaceous gland 19
self-electrolysis 127–9
sexual differentiation 5–8
sexual hair 16–17
shaft, hair 19
shaving 59–64

and electrolysis 61–2
  body 61
  face and neck 60–14
  pros and cons 64
  razors 62–4
shoulder hair 32
social pressure ix, 1–4, 38–9
stress 37
stubble 64

telogen 23, 27
temporary removal 52–89
terminal hair 14
testosterone 16–18, 28, 30, 33–7, 42, 47
  free 33–4
  serum 46
tests, medical 45–6
thigh hair 32
thioglycates 65–6
threading 75
trimming 65
types of hair 14

vellus hair 14
virilization 41

waxing 75–89
  application 76–9
  ingredients 75–6
  side-effects 79
women's hair growth 29–51